"My guru taught if you have spiritual knowledge, you should share it. This is the highest form of charity. Audi Gozlan is sharing the divine knowledge of yoga in the form of this beautiful book he wrote. The knowledge shared in this book comes from Audi's experience and from the depth of his heart. Hopefully, it will find its way into the hearts of those who read it, and help them on the path of yoga. May we all move from the darkness of ignorance to the light of knowledge."

—**Sri Dharma Mittra**, founder of Dharma Yoga and the Dharma Yoga Center NYC, and author of Maha Sadhana: Life of Postures, *Asanas, Yoga Wisdom, Maha Sadhana*

"Audi Gozlan's passionate exploration of Jewish mysticism and yoga that began in his teens informs this exquisitely written book. I found *Kabalah Yoga* profoundly moving, widening the path of Jewish spirituality to embrace the movement and form of yoga postures. If you like to move, as I do, and are inspired by Rumi or Theresa of Avila or Mirabai or the Baal Shem Tov or *A Course in Miracles*, you will keep this book close to your heart. Whatever name you use to call to the Divine, this book will open every shuttered window of your body, mind, and spirit to let the love of the eternal shine through. Gozlan's *Kabalah Yoga* will become a classic of mystical philosophy and practice in all traditions."

—**Amy Weintraub**, founder of LifeForce Yoga, and author of
Yoga for Depression and *Yoga Skills for Therapists*

"Yoga is a dance of body and soul and it belongs to everyone. Although the techniques are universal, we each need to adapt the technology into a system that intimately supports our individual life and value system. This brave book emerges from Audi's many years of personal experience into the depth and mysteries, and invites us into revealing the light that shines in us all."

—**Lorin Roche, PhD**, expert in the field of meditation; author of
Meditation Made Easy, Breath Taking, and *Whole Body Meditations*;
and coauthor of *Meditation Secrets for Women* and *Meditation 24/7*

"Audi Gozlan's unique blend of soul, breath, and body is deeply original and powerful.

His grace in movement, coupled with his belief that self-improvement is within reach for all of us, is infectious, motivating, and a call to action! Over and above the yoga, *Kabalah Yoga* will leave you feeling elated."

—**Moses Znaimer**, founder of ZoomerMedia Limited, and executive
producer of ONE TV

"I believe that yoga is art. I believe that yoga teachers are artists, and that the work that they synthesize and share with the world is a composition; some naturally more unique than others. At our agency, we are blessed to help share and support many yoga artists. I find the way Audi has authentically woven together and presented the ancient wisdom traditions of yoga and Kabalah to be exhilarating: a refreshing, completely new and completely accessible synthesis. I feel that Audi has taken Kabalah Yoga down from the heavens and placed it for us on our yoga mats. For that I give thanks."

—**Ava Taylor,** COO of YAMA Talent

"The world is now more than ever ready for an integration of knowledge with the Sacred. In a world growing of adversarial forces against oneness, it is now time for each of us to embrace the opportunity to 'upward salute' the wisdom that the most gifted rabbis have brought forward to us with ancient Hebrew as a whisper of hope…. Only oneness exists and can be felt when we breathe, relax, and feel. Our potential is released from the mustard seed of our soul's desire to be united with life when we let our bodies flow with the grace in movement aligned with the Hebrew letters. The roots will set you free!

Blessings to my dear friend Audi for writing this book, and who I hold most dear in my heart. You will learn how to feel, move, and flow with the Divine to reawaken your connection to spirit and each other. I pray for every human to read this beautiful book. I am honored and in glory to see it make its way to each of you.

Namaste"

—**Jennifer (Devorah) Buergermeister,** MA, RYS, founder of
Rootism®, The Texas Yoga Association and Conference, and
Jennyoga® (subsidiaries of Breathe the Cure®, Inc.)

"Audi Gozlan has filled this beautiful book with a plethora of wisdom that inspires us to go deeper into our practice of yoga, and bring more awareness of our life and connection to heaven and earth. We are much closer than we think!"

—**Michele Bohbot,** Iyengar certified teacher, LAYT certified yoga
therapist, founder of Bisou Bisou, and founder of Namastday Yoga
Center in Beverly Hills, CA

"It gives me great honor, and my heart immense joy, to share my endorsement for Kabalah Yoga in general, and for Audi's new book. Audi Gozlan's Kabalah Yoga is no less than a stroke of genius. Audi is a soul pioneer, who with great depth of heart, bridges the world of yoga and mystical spirituality. His new book, *Kabalah Yoga*, successfully reveals the sacred beauty of the Divine Spirit that resides in each of us, and lays out a tangible path to bring forth these inner treasures into our lives, and the world. For those of us on a spiritual, heart-centered path who seek for meaning and richness in our inner lives, this is a must-read."

    —**Karen Heaven Claffey**, DOMP, certified Anusara yoga teacher, C-IAYT, E-RYT500

"A humble wise soul
    Audi Gozlan is a keeper of the eternal flame
    A bridge builder who decodes this sacred wisdom of yoga and the Kabalah and makes it accessible for the world to experience and benefit from."

    —**Moses Love**, artist, musician, yoga teacher, and founder of I Love Yoga

"Given so much of what is happening in the world, a practice that fosters inner peace is a key part of wellness. And with his Kabalah Yoga teachings, Audi Gozlan offers precisely this by utilizing an ancient philosophy which is incredibility relevant today. This gentle guru leads you on a journey that unites the body and spirit through mindful movement. It delivers a profound experience unlike any other and forms a pathway to better health and more happiness."

    —**Suzanne Boyd**, editor in chief of *ZOOMER Magazine*

Kabalah YOGA

Embodying the Hidden Power of the Sacred Hebrew Letters

AUDI GOZLAN, RYT

REVEAL PRESS

AN IMPRINT OF NEW HARBINGER PUBLICATIONS

Distributed in Canada by Raincoast Books

Copyright © 2017 by Audi Gozlan
          New Harbinger Publications, Inc.
          5674 Shattuck Avenue
          Oakland, CA 94609
          www.newharbinger.com

Cover design by Amy Shoup

Acquired by Jess O'Brien

Edited by Rona Bernstein

All Rights Reserved

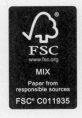 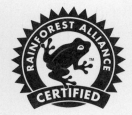

Library of Congress Cataloging-in-Publication Data on file

19   18   17

10   9   8   7   6   5   4   3   2   1   First Printing

I was lucky to have bathed for eighteen years in the sacred light of my root teacher the Rebbe. I am forever grateful to have been able to breathe from his air, learning so much about life, fulfilling dreams, and living our potential. The Rebbe was a great leader not just because his wisdom was powerful but also because when he saw in you a potential, he would bless, motivate, and inspire you to do everything you can to bring it out and shine light and love into our world. Twenty-three years after his passing to higher realms, the voice still reverberates, the face still radiates, and the presence continues to be felt.

I humbly present this manuscript hoping to add a little light, warmth, and inspiration.

CONTENTS

FOREWORD

I first met Audi almost ten years ago in one of my afternoon prana vinyasa flow yoga classes at Sacred Movement in Venice Beach, California. It was a typical diverse gathering of more than eighty souls from every walk of life, Los Angeles being one of the epicenters for the evolution of yoga in the West.

As we started the opening movement meditation, we began to trace with our arms the sound of "Aum." In the power of collective sound, we initiated with "Ahhh" from the roots. We flowed into the sound "Uuuu" in the heart region for the sustaining power of love, and then "Mmnnng," resonating in the crown center.

I noticed Audi, near the arched windows, moving with the sounds in a natural prayer, so connected and expressive with his whole body and soul. When I saw that he was wearing a kippah on his head throughout his practice, I knew that he was drawing from a deeper current. We were destined to connect.

I will never forget the evening, a few years later, when Audi lit with us the Shabbat candles as part of our Friday night teacher training meditation. In the circle, we were a microcosm of the world's spiritual traditions—Jewish, First Nation, Sufi, Muslim, Christian, Buddhist, Shamanic—meeting around the light of the heart.

Audi shared the wisdom of the flame of Shabbat, reminding us that the soul is like a flame, constantly rising higher and connecting to the eternal source of light. Everything that exists in the soul, the inner flame, also exists within the body, the carrier of the flame. When we ignite the internal flame, we are also illuminating our entire self. He then made a prayer and showed us a particular Kabalistic body flow as we all gazed at the flames and began moving our arms from the light and into our hearts to receive the radiating blessings.

Audi eloquently described the significance of the movement, saying it was a way of awakening the fire within our heart and the connection to the light in the soul. He said it was something we can all strive for. At that moment, I saw that Audi's unique talent in bringing his personal devotion to the inner mysteries of life was a gift that could benefit us all.

Now, a decade later, I celebrate the pioneering offering that Audi is bringing out. This book will serve those searching to embody mystical wisdom as well as yoga practitioners who want to deepen their practice. Today, more than ever, is the moment to bathe in the wisdom of the eternal light.

Through his deep understanding of the sacred Hebrew letters and of yoga, Audi is creating a bridge between the ancient wisdoms of Kabalah and of yoga, and he is providing a model of integration for all to benefit from. He is excavating the power of the Kabalah teachings about the body, breath, and soul of the sacred letters, and activating that knowledge directly within the cells of the human body.

Now more than ever, people are seeking greater integration within their own spiritual roots, across wisdom traditions, and within their own embodiment to realize the light of the soul within.

Audi is an artist, scholar, yoga practitioner, explorer, and true pioneer. With the gift of this book, he is taking us into a path of feeling much more in our movement and breath. Kabalah Yoga encourages us to search inward and be the vessel that holds our soul flame, shining and elevating everything.

May all who drink from this treasure of wisdom Audi is sharing with us be nourished, awakened, and illuminated within.

May Audi continue to be a vessel for the blessings and teachings of his ancestors, and particularly for the lineage of his root teacher, the Rebbe.

May we all realize the *neshimah* (breath) that is breathing us all. May we realize our *ko-ach* (full potential) as we connect to the *ein sof* (eternal light) that embraces all life.

Infinite Blessings,
ShalOM,

Shiva Rea
Humaliwu New Moon

INTRODUCTION

I am happy to share with you a sacred dimension in the practice of yoga. We are all unique in the way our body energetically moves and dances with the soul to bring us life and creative expression. We are all moving through different levels of being in the flow of life as we develop wisdom.

The practice of yoga gives us the opportunity to evolve, each one of us at our own pace, through newer levels to reach higher vibrations and states of being. Kabalah provides us with the spiritual tools to grow deeper in body and soul, and when practiced with yoga, we can experience a greater feeling of harmony and peace, *shalom*.

In many ways, we are spiritual gardeners, constantly planting new seeds on our path of life. The ones that we nurture are those that we will grow into, and those will become our destiny. We all share the desire to grow into our best self by reaching for our dreams and potential.

From the moment we are born, the soul grows in us together with the body, energizing the mind, the heart, and all of our qualities and reactions, creating every thought, word, and action. Our soul and body were meant to be one, and the more this alignment is made, the deeper will our inner and outer being be united in harmony.

Everything that exists in the soul also exists within the body. The Divine exists deep inside our bones, our blood, and our emotional and mental framework. Our body is the temple, the sacred space that shelters our soul and allows our inner light to shine.

What Is Kabalah Yoga?

Kabalah Yoga is practiced by moving the body into the sacred shapes, *otiot*, using the Hebrew letters as templates to help us tap into the essence and arouse deep feelings and intentions of the heart.

Kabalah is a wisdom that encourages us to search inward, reach deeply within, and discover ourselves from inside out. It is about living now in our potential and assuming our divine role in this world by developing both our physical and our spiritual selves. Everything in this world has a spark of light inside of it.

Because we have a piece of the Divine within, in the form of our soul that keeps our life flame burning, we can elevate everything in this world and help it reveal its own light. You are here on Earth because you matter and can make a difference if you allow your inner light to shine.

Tapping into the essence of life is dependent upon our efforts in moving inward into the soul and entering into our true inner feelings, the *kavana* of the heart, as the soul and body begin to dance. *Kavana* is a soulful experience that we all have at some point in life. In Hebrew, *kavana* also means "to direct" and refers to the direction of the heart as we grow more inward. It can be in the form of a prayer or spiritual experience that brings us out of our limitations or a powerful chant that lifts our spirit. Such a moment can be as simple as a peaceful walk in nature or gazing at a sunset as cool air blows on our face. In all of these, our experiences are felt deeply. If we are not in tune or are disconnected with our now, then seeing and enjoying the many blessings of life will be difficult. Kabalah and yoga are ways that help us appreciate life more fully and taste the sweet juice of essence that is often concealed in our life experiences.

Kabalah in Hebrew means "to receive" and refers to our ability to be receivers of light. *Yoga* in Sanskrit means "union" and refers to the connection of the inner and outer body.

A principal teaching in Kabalah is the concept known as *orot-ve'keilim*, "lights and vessels." Every form of light needs a vessel in order to shine, and each vessel needs light to exist. The light and vessel are so intimate with one another that when the vessel is either revealing or concealing, it is doing the light good.

Neither a light nor a vessel could exist or have a purpose if one were missing from the other. Together, the light and the vessel form a reality that manifests a physical existence to carry divine light.

In the practice of yoga, the body can connect to the soul if we develop deep feelings, *kavana*, that grow from the essence, also known in yoga as *bhava*. In Sanskrit, *bhava* means "emotion, feeling, or state of body and mind." In Buddhism, *bhava* refers to "infinite states of being." *Bha-va* in Hebrew means "entering deeply within."

In Kabalah, *kavana* is the energy that rises from the soul from an open heart that produces intention. This intention makes our service in this world warmer, powerful, and meaningful. It is leading from the heart and soul as we bring our entire self into whatever action we do. *Kavana* exists deeply in our experiences. It is the intention of being now in the moment in mind, body, and soul. It is creating a space to feel free, let go, and visualize a prayer flourishing from our inner self. It is the force behind any thought, word, or action intended to make a difference and transform us. *Kavana* is often felt in movement, music, art, prayer, and meditation. But it can also be experienced in any situation where we become one with the moment being created.

Kavana, "intention," in yoga becomes a tool to fully benefitting from the postures. We can do yoga by awakening the energy of deep inner feelings and start to irrigate the soil of our soul by cultivating greater awareness and depth.

Practicing Kabalah Yoga

From the moment we roll out our mat or practice yoga directly on the Earth, the energy below us becomes the soil upon which our practice will bear fruits. As we settle down on our mat and begin to breathe with more awareness, the mat becomes our terrain from where we will cultivate the seeds of our practice that will bear fruits to savor during the flow, and more importantly after the practice is complete. Like a tree, we have roots, a body, and branches, and can bear fruits. Have you ever observed how a tree grows?

As a seed is planted in the ground, it immediately begins to develop a relationship with the soil, air, water, and sun. The ground offers the seed a platform from which it can rise. Air provides oxygen, water gives nourishment, and the sun is the enlightenment from which the seed finds inspiration to emerge. The seed is in its full *kavana* as it comfortably cuddles into the sacred space created for its growth.

As it sprouts, the seed suddenly shatters and loses itself entirely. If the seed had a mind, it would certainly think that its life were over, that it had been betrayed. Then, at the very moment the seed loses everything of its tiny shell-body, the roots begin to form, reaching deep into the Earth. The sprout rises from the Earth. The roots develop a spine, a central channel for life to flow into, and slowly its new body begins to take shape.

Our practice of yoga can be that of gardening the seeds of our soul. How we choose to begin a practice will be the stage of planting seeds onto the mat, and what is important is the *kavana*, the intention we wish to cultivate. As we begin to move our body into a sequence of various poses, we have available our inner water of wisdom, our air of breath, and our sun, the light of our heart, to irrigate the seeds of our soul and move into the soil of awareness. The energy that blossoms through our practice and how it changes us will be the fruits we will enjoy from our yoga.

The idea of connecting Kabalah and yoga is based on the intention of cultivating the seeds of our yoga practice so they bear the fruits of our soul that we may savor. By moving the body with awareness of the shapes of the letters, we embrace their energy and great wisdom that has existed since the beginning of time—a wisdom that empowers, heals, and enhances our entire life.

Kabalah Yoga is a *hatha* practice with the awareness that the postures are powerful tools that help you journey deeply inward toward your essence by discovering your soul in the body of the postures. *Hatha* is a Sanskrit term that means *ha*, "the sun," and *tha*, "the moon," and refers to the union of two opposites. While Kabalah maybe compared to the light of your soul that shines in you, yoga is similar to the moon and your body is the vessel that carries this light. Kabalah Yoga implies that the practice is intended to bring harmony between your body and soul by cultivating yourself inwardly and outwardly.

Kabalah Yoga is the fruit that grew from seeds I planted early in my life and have ever since been irrigating. My body has served me as the ground through which I could find the expression of my soul.

My Journey

I have been blessed to be surrounded by spiritual gardeners, who during my lifetime have taught me how to cultivate the fruits of my soul and prepare the soil of awareness for my body to be a vessel. I was born in Montreal to a Moroccan-Jewish family that immigrated from Israel in the 1960s. Although we were not very religious, we lived in a Hassidic neighborhood where I attended a Yeshiva, an all-boys school that taught both the mystical practice and the spiritual life of the Torah. In Yeshiva, I discovered ancient texts that spoke to me. I learned about the secrets of the soul, life, and the purpose of existence, and that the Creator was a great artist. I contemplated on living a meaningful life and was discovering that I had artistic talent.

I have loved to draw ever since I was a child. Like many kids, I had my colored pencils and sketching pad that I carried with me wherever I went, hoping to see something interesting to draw. The energy of drawing has allowed me to grow closer to my dreams and enter into a subconscious state where I can imagine a situation altogether different from what I am living. My passion for drawing has always been very special to me, something I continue to do to this very day.

At eight years old, I had the great honor of meeting the Lubavitcher Rebbe Menachem Mendel Schneerson, who became the most important spiritual influence of my life. For a long time, I was only interested in drawing the Rebbe. Like no other teacher I ever had, the Rebbe, as we call him, opened my heart in such a way that I was able to bear many fruits of the mind, heart, body, and soul. Throughout my life, the Rebbe inspired me to go deeper into myself, to envision, to draw, to meditate, to become a lawyer, and to develop Kabalah Yoga.

Meditation, like drawing, helps us get out of the box and into the subconscious as we come closer to our dreams. Meditation is the art of focusing the mind on something positive that will energize the mind-and-body connection. It is also a way to transcend the never-ending flow of thoughts that occupy our brain. In yoga, this is described as controlling breath, or *prana*, to reach deeper into our inner world and gain more awareness. When we reach this point of awareness, we are free to be without any other thought but to simply be in our breath.

At age fifteen, I had my first meditative experience with my then best friend, Yehuda, with whom I share the same Hebrew name. He often traveled to India with his family to be with their guru, Swami G. in Kulu, Valley of the Gods, and shared the Swami's teachings with me.

My time with Yehuda was always precious. Our thirst for knowing the unknown and dipping into the mystery of life kept our bond deep and strong. The heights we reached spiritually sometimes seemed too much for us as high school boys, though these were exciting moments, for we were curious and wanting to touch the Divine. We learned the *Tanya*, an esoteric work authored in the nineteenth century by Kabalist and Hassidic master Rabbi Schneur Zalman of Liadi, Russia, founder of the Habad movement over 250 years ago and predecessor of the Rebbe.

Yehuda shared with me *pranic* breathing. Slowly through breathing exercises, art, meditation, and the study of mysticism, I began to develop awareness, breath control, and better focus. These lessons were the seeds that years later would attract me to the practice of yoga and the development of Kabalah Yoga.

As I got older, I continued to feed my interest in the esoteric, reading works that touched the mystical, including the *Torah*, *Talmud*, Kabalah, *Book of Prophets*, and Midrashim. I embraced the writings of my teacher the Rebbe, hoping to grasp something deeper and allow the light of Kabalah to shine on everything I learned. Often, I felt like I was trying to drink all the water in a river with a spoon, but as I grew into the heart and soul of Kabalah, every drop of wisdom quenched my thirst and opened me to new levels of awareness. I nourished my hunger for intellectual stimulation. My first degree was in political science, focusing on philosophy and studying the works of Machiavelli, Aristotle, Plato, Socrates, Nietzsche, and other philosophers. With the blessings of the Rebbe, I went on to study law and became a lawyer.

I was always an active person. In my younger years, I played various sports year-round, including baseball and football during the summer and ice hockey in the winter. In my twenties, I took up body building, biking, and jogging. The more active I was, the more I became aware of my body and the need to move in a way that would take me inward. I began taking *hatha* and hot yoga classes weekly. I was hooked. I was finally moving my body in a way that was touching me deeply.

Little by little, I was beginning to see my body as a sacred dwelling for my soul.

The Discovery

"There is nothing new under the sun."

—Kohelet 1:9

"Each thing ever found and will be found, has existed since the beginning."

—Rashi, Genesis 1:1; *Bereishit Raba*

One evening while preparing for the weekly talk on Kabalah that I offered, I was flipping through some sacred books and opened the mystical text *Keter Shem Tov Hashalem*, a compilation of teachings of the holy Baal Shem Tov, the founder of the Hassidic movement in the 1700s. I was looking for deeper understanding about the Hebrew letters, as the theme of the class was about the secrets of the Hebrew letters. As I leafed through the pages, I came across the following teaching: "Each Hebrew letter had a soul, breath, and body."

What did this mean? It sounded more like yoga to me than Kabalah! I began to ponder this teaching. My mind was working hard, going from imagination to meditation and to yoga.

The Hebrew letters are like the human body (*guf* in Hebrew) because they have arms, a spine, and legs. The breath (*neshima*) is the energy that fills the world (*olam*) of the letter, just as an aura exists in each person. The soul (*neshamah*) is the essence of the letter, the divine (*elokut*) spark that gives life to the body. The soul is revealed when good intention fills us with inspiration and lifts our life to the highest spiritual level.

From this moment of inspiration, I began to dream of the shapes of each letter as movements of the body. I was shaping into poses with a feeling that the body was divine if I would allow myself to flow with sacred intentions. I searched in Kabalah, the Torah, and *The Talmud* for anything written about the Hebrew letters. I began to see from the perspective of the Baal Shem Tov, realizing that most of the ancient teachings in Kabalah come down to an understanding of the Hebrew letters in body, breath, and soul. I took out my sketching pad and pencils and began drawing the Hebrew letters as body shapes.

Then, one day while in a *hatha* yoga class, we were doing the Warrior II Pose, and it all came together. As I stood strong, with my feet planted on the mat and my arms extended outward, I suddenly had an awareness that I was taking on the shape of the Hebrew letter *Alef* (A). This was my aha moment that would change what I understood about the Hebrew letters and yoga. Experiencing something is always more powerful than just thinking of something. An artist can have a masterpiece in his mind, but if it stays in the realm of thought, his painting is worthless. The teaching of the Baal Shem Tov that every letter has a soul, body, and breath was something I was finally experiencing in the Warrior II Pose. The *Alef* was my entrance into a whole new understanding of Kabalah and yoga that has transformed my life.

"It is through your body that you realize you are a spark of divinity."

—B. K. S. Iyengar

Once I started looking for the sacred shapes in yoga postures, I began to see more and more of the Hebrew characters that I had been meditating upon for so many years. Each Hebrew letter became my template for matching various postures into one similar shape. This five-thousand-year-old biblical dialect used in learning, praying, reading, and writing now became a powerful language for the body to embrace. Yoga was the vessel for moving my body into the Hebrew letters and connecting to their soul, body, and breath.

My studies in Kabalah became deeper. I was learning in order to share the sacred wisdom so it could be applied to the practice of yoga. At the same time, I was intensively practicing yoga daily and went on to study in depth in *hatha*, Anusara, and Prana Vinyasa. I have learned so much from all my yoga teachers and colleagues, including Hart Lazer in *hatha*, Karen Claffey in Anusara, and my wife Karen in alignment and my first taste of flow yoga.

In 2008, I met Shiva Rea, founder of Prana Vinyasa, in Venice Beach, California, and was captivated by her passion and grace. She was teaching yoga as a sacred movement. I am grateful to have learned so much from Shiva and her teachings on Prana Vinyasa. She is the seasoning that brought out the taste of my practice of yoga. Shiva inspired me to deepen through *bhava*, "inner feelings," and to see that postures could be grouped together according to their shapes. Some *asanas*, she explained, "are closely related like siblings, while others are connected like cousins." Some postures are necessary for entering a peak posture, while others are there to support the body before or after a posture. On this basis, I have grouped poses into families for each Hebrew letter corresponding to their shape and energy. Kabalah Yoga as a method of movement is a work in progress because there exists an infinite reservoir of wisdom to be explored and more possible postures for each letter, which I hope to share with you at a later time.

The Hebrew Letters as Sacred Shapes

Kabalah has a great secret about the Hebrew letters unknown to most people. The mystics say the sacred shapes, *otiot* in Hebrew, are codes within each form of life, creating and emanating them out of nothingness. Without these shapes, life would cease to exist. Kabalah tells us that during the seven days of creation, these sacred shapes were used as the Creator's tools to make the world. By combining the letters into meaningful words, mantras infused with intention and deep breath, the words uttered powerfully bore fruits as they penetrated the very fabric of creation. The secret of the Hebrew letters is that they are the templates for all the physical realities they represent and constantly create and renew all forms of life.

Kabalah explains that Adam, the first man in the Garden of Eden, received the secret wisdom of *Leshon Hakodesh,* or "sacred tongue," directly from the Creator. He observed the unique breath and movement of each animal, bird, and species and named it by combining specific letters according to its essence and nature. We hear Adam in the Bible, conversing in this divine language with the Creator and Eve, his female partner. Even the infamous snake in the Garden of Eden spoke in this mystical way to Eve.

During the first thousand years of creation, all beings spoke the sacred tongue as the family of Adam and Eve began to grow. However, because humans brought darkness upon the Earth, the world ceased being the paradise it was intended to be, and the sacred tongue was being forgotten.

The sages explain that the story of the failed coup of the Tower of Babel 1,656 years after Adam is the turning point in history that gave birth to the many languages of the world. The Kabalah of the sacred shapes, however, had been kept a secret and carefully taught only to a select few—the most pious and purest of souls from each generation.

According to tradition, Adam taught the secrets of the Hebrew letters to Hanoch, his great grandson, and to Metuselah, the grandfather of Noah. These two masters then revealed the wisdom to Noah, who taught it to his son Shem, the first Kabalah master. Shem then transmitted the teaching of the shapes to Abraham, who sometime in 1700 BC (eighteenth century BCE) compiled the first Kabalah text, *Sefer Yetsirah, The Book of Shapes,* also known as *The Otiot of*

Abraham. Incidentally, this is the same period in which the *Vedas* were being composed by the children of Brahma in India.

Abraham and the Hebrew Letters

"The secret sacred shapes were revealed to none other than Abraham."

—Midrash, *Pirkei d'Rabbi Eliezer*

Abraham continued the transmission by teaching the secrets to his son Isaac, who then taught it to Jacob, who shared the knowledge with his children. Eventually the wisdom reached Moses, who used the sacred language to teach the Torah to the Hebrew people God had liberated from slavery in Egypt and brought to the promised land.

In my research, I discovered that there is yet another side to Abraham's transmission of the secret wisdom of the Hebrew letters. In chapter 25 of Genesis, the Torah says that following the death of Sarah, Abraham married a woman named Ketura. She was also known as Hagar, the servant of Sarah and the mother of Ishmael, Abraham's first born. She was the daughter of Pharaoh, king of Egypt, who chose to be a maidservant to the great Abraham rather than be a princess.

Ketura bore six other sons to Abraham. They were named Zimran, Yokshan, Madan, Midan, Yishbak, and Shuach. The Midrash tells us that their names reflected their deeds. For example, Zimran is singer to deities, and Yokshan is drummer to deities. They were the younger brothers of Ishmael and Isaac. While Isaac remained in Canaan, Ishmael was sent by Abraham to the Desert of Paran, which spreads from Assyria to Egypt.

Zimran, Yokshan, Madan, Midan, Yishbak, and Shuach were sent to the "land of the East," the biblical reference for India. The Torah tells us that Abraham sent them to the East with precious gifts, *matanot*, described by the sages as mystical secrets related to the cosmos of creation. According to Rashi, the most important Torah commentator of the twelfth century, among the gifts that Abraham gave them were the healing powers to overcome *tumas* or *tamas*, the Hindu word for "darkness." Behind the letters that spell *tumas* in Hebrew are allusions to these healing gifts, notably *Tet* ("karma"), *Vav* ("balance"), *Mem* ("space"), and *Heih* ("breath").

The Talmud tells us that aside from *The Book of Shapes*, Abraham also authored a second book consisting of four hundred chapters covering worshipping practices, which was also among the gifts he gave to his children. With these gifts, the sons of Abraham began their spiritual quest in India.

According to fifteenth-century Kabalist Menashe Ben Israel in his book *Nishmat Chayim, "Living Soul,"* the sons were initially known in India as the Abrahmans, the children of the famous Abraham. As they integrated into this new land, they became known as the Brahmans, important priests, as they spread the teachings of their father in India, where Abraham became known as Brahma and his wife Sarah as Sarahsvati.

Inspired by Abraham's teachings on creation, the Brahmans composed the sacred *Vedas* (meaning the "knowledge" in both Sanskrit and Hebrew), where yoga, "to bond," is mentioned for the first time in the *Rig Veda* (one of the four *Vedas*). It is not clear whether the word "yoga" was meant to be a form of movement or even of meditation. It appears that "yoga" is meant to refer to harmony, stillness, and unity of the inner and outer self. The more we look inward beyond the layers of life, the closer we will come to our essence.

I believe that Abraham shared with all his children the teachings of the soul, body, and breath through the secrets of the shapes of the letters. While Isaac received this through the mystical teachings of Kabalah, the Brahmans were given the gifts of translating the letters as *asanas*, shapes in yoga; meditation, *dhyana*; and breath, *prana*.

Sacred Wisdom

Early Jewish mystical works deal extensively with the symbolism and secret meaning of the Hebrew letters. Following Abraham's *Sefer Yetsirah*, further teachings on Kabalah were compiled in the writings of the sage Akivah (c. 700) in his *Otiot d'Rabbi Akivah* (c. 700), and the *Alphabet of Ben Sira* (*Alphabetum Siracidis*, c. 700). The most well-known works are *Pirkei d'Rabbi Eliezer, Book of Razi'el, Book of Bahir,* the *Heikhalot* writings, *Sefer Temunah, Shi'ur Komah, Harba d'Moshe,* and *Sefer Ha-Yashar.* The sacred shapes as spiritual states of creation are discussed in the *Zohar*, in the writings of Moses Cordovero, and in *Shi'ur Komah.* Also important are the sections of *The Talmud* and the Midrashim that discuss the esoteric.

The Midrash Talpiot states that while some letters have a feminine shape, others are masculine. The meaning of this gendering in the text is that some shapes, like the *Alef* (as in Warrior II Pose), represent strength and power, which is characterized as a male energy. Other letters that open the heart, as in the letter *Beit* (Crescent Moon Pose) or *Cheit* (Wheel Pose), are said to represent female energy.

Another important source is thirteen-century Spanish Kabalist Abraham Abulafia, author of various meditative works on the Hebrew letters as channels of energy. It is related that Abulafia had a close student artist named Nathan Shem Tov from Lyon, France, who drew the Hebrew letters as energetic body postures according to his master Abulafia's mystical teachings. Below is a drawing of the *Alef* shaped as a human body assuming the Warrior II by the artist Nathan made over eight hundred years ago.

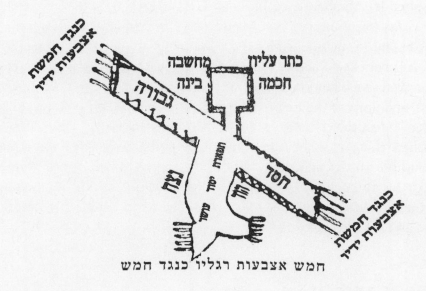

Sefer Sha'arei Tsedek, compiled by Amnon Gross, published by the Beit Hasefarim of the University of Jerusalem, Israel, 2008.

Who This Book Is For

This book is meant for anyone searching to live a more meaningful life by deepening their presence. Whether you are a beginner or an advanced yoga practitioner, learning the sacred shapes will deepen your practice of yoga and bring new light into your flow.

Kabalah is designed to guide us into wholeness, authentic connection, and honest reflection into our spirituality. Yoga is an Eastern holistic approach to our health and happiness that teaches us how to reach deeply into the body and inner energy through the power of breath, *prana*, or *ruach* in Hebrew.

Kabalah Yoga offers ancient wisdom that benefits our physical practice of yoga and supports our spiritual growth. It is for someone who is new to yoga or who has been practicing for a long time, whether a student or teacher of yoga. It is also meant for anyone searching for practical spirituality that touches the body as deeply as it reaches into the soul.

The sacred shapes are rich with meaning, energy, and guidance for life. This book is divided and organized according to the order of the twenty-two Hebrew letters. Each chapter offers a lesson on the Hebrew letter according to Kabalah as well as cues and guidelines to posture into the shapes according to yoga. Each chapter includes the letter's corresponding English letter, the Hebrew letter's numerical value, and a discussion about the letter's soul, breath, and body. The "Soul" section covers the meaning of the letter, the "Breath" section includes the pulsation in each movement and discusses the intentions derived from the letter, and the "Body" section defines the guidelines for how to come into the poses and embrace the energy of each shape.

Of the twenty-two Hebrew letters, five have an alternative shape. These five are *Khaf (K)*, *Mem (M)*, *Nun (N)*, *Peih (P, F)*, and *Tsadik (Ts)*.

As well, the names of some of the sacred shapes have alternative pronunciations. *Beit (B)* can be pronounced as "veit," *Khaf (K)* as "chaf," *Peih (P)* as "feih," *Shin (Sh)* as "sien," and *Tav (T)* as "sav." Mystically, these differences represent various ways their energy is revealed. This book will refer to the letters by their original pronunciations.

How to Use This Book

Each Hebrew letter has a unique shape that represents the way its energy flows. The shape is the space we form with our body for light to shine internally. In putting into practice the sacred shapes, it is good to go through the letters one at a time to appreciate the deep meaning of each.

Familiarize yourself with the yoga postures that correspond to each letter. The yoga postures in this book are grouped according to their shape and resemblance to the Hebrew letters as templates. Once you recognize the shape your body assumes, you can begin to assimilate postures that fall in the same family into a flow that draws the body and soul connection closer.

By using the ABCs of each letter, you will be able to create flows that form words and even your own name. You can also flow according to numbers that correspond to each of the letter values.

An inspiring thought about the Hebrew letters from Akivah, author of *Otiot d'Rabbi Akivah*, begins each chapter. Akivah was an awesome being, whose story is discussed further in the conclusion. He was the one who revealed to the world *Sefer Yetsirah*, *The Book of Shapes of Abraham* and many of the secrets concerning the unique image and energy of each letter. I cite him throughout the book because of his simple and yet powerful wisdom that humanizes the deep teachings of Kabbalah on the Hebrew letters.

Each chapter is divided into three parts: "Soul" (intention), "Breath" (pulsation), and "Body" (shape) guided in the spirit of Prana Vinyasa that will bring you into a sacred practice to bring harmony and alignment into your outer and inner selves.

Soul is the essence of the Hebrew letter that reveals deep intentions that inspire the movement of our breath and body. The soul of the letter is associated with its wisdom expressed through an intention. Intention is manifested in deep feelings that can be felt in the body through breath. The soul of each letter is the wisdom behind the shapes and how we can embrace it as we come into each template pose and experience intention in our breath and body. The soul awareness opens the path to devotional feelings that induce a deep connection with our inner being. As we see ourselves from the essence, through cultivating *kavana*, "deep feelings," our awareness in yoga becomes more powerful.

Breath is the pulsation of the inhale and exhale within the body as the first movement of the posture. Breath is the vital force that pulsates in every organ, limb, cell, and molecule, and is the closest union we have with the creator. As the body moves into the shape of each letter with intention, we become the embodiment of its energy. We connect to our inner feelings through breath. When we are happy, we breathe with expanded lungs, and when we are worried, our breath is shortened. We need to breathe slower, deeper, and with more awareness. Awareness of our breath will affect the energy that causes our lungs to contract, our heart to beat, and our blood to flow through the body.

Our breath can move us deeper within, beyond the flesh and bones. If we breathe with awareness, then our breath becomes the vehicle that carries our *kavana*, deep feelings that stem from our essence. When we open our heart with *kavana*, we are directing our practice of yoga into such feelings as love, compassion, understanding, joy, and happiness. Breath is the bridge that carries our intention from the essence into the movement of the body.

The "Body" section explains the movement of the yoga pose so you can embrace the shape of the letter. Each letter posture has a unique shape that represents the way its energy flows. The body of the posture is the vessel that becomes the movement of the inner energy of the soul created in the body through inner feelings, *kavana*, and spread into your body through your breath.

⌇⌇⌇⌇⌇⌇⌇⌇⌇⌇⌇⌇⌇⌇

With the teachings of the body, breath, and soul of each posture, your yoga practice can become a powerful tool in positively influencing your personal life and the world at large. I share with you the Hebrew letters as templates to your practice of yoga that will help you draw deeper into the essence of your flow and arouse deep feelings of the heart, and a clear mind, to reach into your potential.

I begin with the first sacred shape, *Alef (A)*, the master warrior and symbol of union between the universe and you. The *Alef* bridges all differences and everything inside and outside of us, and awakens within a feeling of oneness. As you study the *Alef* and all the letters that follow, welcome the energy of each of the sacred shapes of yoga as a way of living, thinking, being, reviving, healing, connecting, and smiling.

Enjoy the journey!

ShalOM

Audi

CHAPTER 1

ALEF: Oneness

Pose: Warrior II

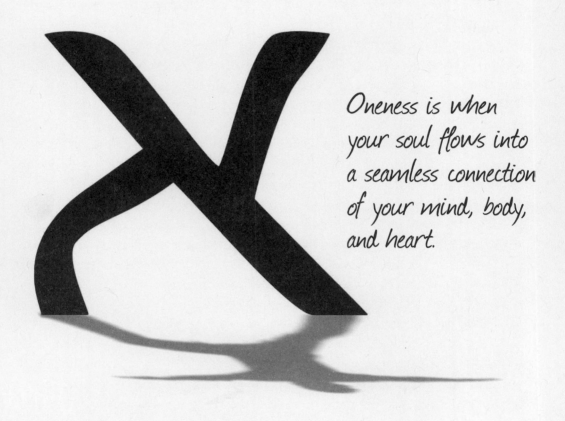

Oneness is when your soul flows into a seamless connection of your mind, body, and heart.

The *Alef*, the first letter of the Hebrew alphabet, corresponds to the English letters *A*, *E*, *O*, and *U* and has a numerical value of 1.

Soul

Alef: Alef rishon, Vehu Alouf Acharon. "The *Alef* is the first and eternal master."

—Akivah

Since I was a young boy, the letter *Alef* has fascinated me. Aside from being the first Hebrew letter I learned in kindergarten, corresponding to the letter A, it was also the first shape I learned when I was taught to spell my name, Audi, in Hebrew. *Alef* has the value of one. The letter *Alef* is made of three lines: two short lines, one above and the other below and a longer line in between them, holding the two shorter ones together.

My father once told me that he named me Audi because when he was a young man serving in the Israeli army in the 1950s, he was a big fan of Audie Murphy. Audie was one of America's most decorated soldiers, who fought in World War II and then became a famous actor starring in many western movies. This thought of Audie Murphy always inspired me to be a soldier of life, to have the courage to battle my own little wars, and to express myself as I am, Audi.

As I grew older and began to understand more deeply the Hebrew language in reading and writing, I realized that interpretation was essential not only to understanding the meaning of the word, but also its energy. The Hebrew letters are energy channels that we can tap into by connecting to their breath and light. Because they symbolize letters and numbers, many meanings can be associated with each letter, especially when combined with other letters (known in Hebrew as *gematria*). When the Hebrew letters make up a word, the word also receives its power by the letters' definitions and implications. This is especially relevant if it is a word that affects you personally, such as your name.

"Audi" in Hebrew means "to praise and show gratitude." In Latin, "Audi" also means "to be heard," as in the term *audi alteram partem*, meaning "Everyone has the right to be heard." The letters that spell "Audi" in Hebrew and their meanings are *Alef (A)*, one; *Vav (U)*, alignment; *Dalet (D)*, freedom; and *Yud (I)*, humility. Because these letters are the same as the sacred shapes that brought creation, they too carry hidden energies that we can tap into.

When I looked into the meanings of the letters, I realized that the name Audi, which I have been carrying throughout my life and have been called by it by thousands if not more people, has deeply affected me personally.

The sages say that that the world was created through sacred words, or *mantras*, being repeated until the things they meant came to be. According to Kabalah, because you are called by your name, your name will touch you deeply and affect your energy. "Audi," for example, has taught me to be thankful for all the blessings in my life, to be strong and face challenges, to grow from inside, and to live my dreams.

When you learn about the sacred shapes that spell your name, you will discover a great deal of personal wisdom about yourself that will help you understand your spiritual connection, and what needs to be cultivated in body and soul. I discovered later that Audie Murphy, like myself, also had a middle name. His was Leon, and mine is Yehuda, both meaning "lion," to be grounded and strong.

The Letter

The *Alef* reveals that within each of us is a divine light that embraces all of existence. Your soul is that light, known as *ore* in Hebrew, and comes from the Creator's light. Because you share the same light, you are one with the Creator. The Creator is everywhere, and although we may not see it as we see the physical world, still, we *can* see with the eye of the soul. As part of your human qualities, you have the ability to look inward and see from deep within. This inner vision can be reached if you clear your mind and open your heart to what is real and meaningful to you. You may say to yourself, "Easier said than done!" This is true. However, what is also true is that with some effort, you can begin to see the inside as you see outside by practicing looking inward.

To be in the flow of the *Alef*, your body and soul must move together as one, physically and spiritually. Your body needs your soul as much as your soul needs your body. To be in the rhythm of oneness, neither the body nor the soul can be ignored. While the body has its needs for survival, the soul too has its essentials. If we deny one, then we are also denying the other. We cannot ignore the body's needs to eat, sleep, move, and just be. Nor can we put aside the soul's expression through breath, silence, meditation, and creative expression. If we listen carefully to the body and soul, we will start to hear a soft voice coming from deep within asking for attention. Your body and soul are telling you to move them together in a rhythmic flow of oneness.

Oneness should not be confused with singleness, because singleness involves constantly moving our attention from the demands of the body to those of the soul. Some days we spend our time nourishing the soul by acts of kindness and compassion. On other days, we are more materially inclined, more physical about ourselves, and more selfish in ways where we are only interested in "me." Ideally, we should be both constantly and simultaneously focusing on the soul and body, bringing the two together as one. The tension between the two is released not by choosing one over the other, but by using the two to fulfill the very same purpose, spiritualizing the material and materializing the spiritual. Without the body, the soul could never fulfill its mission on Earth, and without the soul, the body could never have the focus and awareness it needs in its journey through life. Together, the body and soul form the space necessary for the energy of this union to be translated into breath and into movement.

The *Alef* symbolizes the essence of your soul, its vitality, and its inner light wanting to shine through you. The soul is in your body as it is in your heart and mind. Your feet need your soul as much as your hands and brain do. The soul finds expression in every part of you, but particularly within your breath. Breath is the sign of life and proof that the soul is in the body. In Hebrew, the word for soul, *neshamah* ("divine light within"), is the same word as breath, *neshimah* ("divine breath"), pronounced slightly differently but contain the same letters. This connection reminds us how we really are one with the Creator, deeply bonded through our common breath, the most powerful way we unite to the source of life.

〜〜〜〜〜〜〜〜〜〜

Take a moment to focus on your breath. Sit comfortably, with your spine long, and relax your shoulders. Inhale and exhale from your nose. Inhale, and listen to the soft sound of your breath. Exhale, and release any tension and stiffness in your body. Inhale, and notice your breath as it comes in. Exhale, and notice it again. Repeat a few times and allow each round to bring you deeper into the sound and feeling of your breath. Breathing with awareness is the best way to cultivate your search for oneness.

〜〜〜〜〜〜〜〜〜〜

A story is told of a rabbi who wanted to teach his son about the deeper meaning of life. He called one of his best students into his study room to discuss a proposition. The rabbi said, "You have a duty, and I have a duty. Your duty is to support your family, and mine is to provide my son with an education. Let us work together to fulfill these duties. You will teach my son, and I will compensate you so that you can support your family." The rabbi then told his student how to teach his son: "Begin with the letter *Alef,* for it is a point above, a point below, and a diagonal line in between, all of which make up One." The rabbi wanted the teacher to begin with the image of the *Alef* because this shape contains wisdom not only to be acquired as a child, but also to carry on throughout life.

The *Alef,* a symbol of oneness and unity, is the first letter I discovered many years ago that resembled the Warrior II Pose. Our legs represent the Earth, and our upper body is the Creator within, represented by extended arms of the *Alef,* reaching for the sky. The line in the middle of the *Alef* represents the heart, our gateway to the one light.

The sages explain that the diagonal line of the letter *Alef* is a window that we look through to see the eternal light, and in turn the eternal light looks through that window and sees us. The diagonal line stemming from the heart is also compared to a spiritual mirror that allows us to see our inner selves. When you look into the divine mirror, you see a light that is a reflection of an infinite you. The remarkable feature of a mirror is that when you look into it, not only do you see yourself, but also everything that is before, behind, below, and above you. This is also true with a centered heart that navigates all energies into each part of the body.

The *Alef* is the inner voice of courage that whispers into our ears, to perceive and see the infinite light. When the Creator looks into the mirror, he sees you, a divine image of his being. Think of your heart as a spiritual mirror for you to find what is deep inside your body and soul. Nourish yourself with truth (*emet*), love (*ahava*), unity (*achdut*), and oneness (*echad*), each of which also stems from the *Alef*.

Breath: Energetic Shape and Intention

The kavanas *of the* Alef *are feelings of wholeness, oneness, harmony, unity, light, and fire in the heart.*

The *Alef* requires focus, harmony, groundedness, and strength. The inhale is at the lifting and coiling of the center of the pelvic floor above the thighs. The exhale is on the rooting down through your legs as your feet connect to the Earth energetically. The inhale is also the opening of the arms from the heart radiating with light. The exhale is the gathering as you draw the hands, for example, into the heart.

When shaping your body into the *Alef,* your legs become the symbol of the Earth. The more rooted you are into the four corners of your feet with your weight moving from the pelvis to the knee, such as in Warrior II or Side Angle Pose, the higher you will rise toward heaven. Your heart is the window for seeing the resemblance of your body and soul rooted in the one light. With your heart you can navigate deep feelings and intention through cultivating *kavana* based on learning the various meanings of the *Alef* to inspire you to go deeper.

There are a few variations of the *Alef* we can assume: Warrior II, Reverse Warrior, Extended Side Angle, and Extended Triangle. Each of these poses, when practiced with awareness of the *Alef,* brings out *Alef's* energy through its unique shape and benefits to the body. The main pose is Warrior II, the pose that unites us to all directions, bringing the body into a sense of oneness and unity.

When you extend your arms out, imagine that you are gathering the sparks of light that fill the entire space around you. Through deep, energetic breath, you can draw this feeling into the heart.

Extended Side Angle Pose draws its energy from the core. The heart receives from the core its power and shines by extending one arm over the head. The inhale is at the stretching of your arm into the sky and over your head. The exhale is at the rooting down of your hips and feet.

Extended Triangle Pose symbolizes the *Alef* radiating energy from the Earth into the heart, and consciously extending the arm toward the sky. The inhale is at the stretching of your arm toward the sky. The exhale is at the grounding of your legs. The triangle reminds us that we are always connected to the Earth and sky, and with an energetic heart, we can shine.

Keep the *Alef* in mind as you go through the family of variations pertaining to Warrior II. *Alef* is the letter that receives light directly from the *ein sof*, the "eternal light," passing it along to the other letters and imbuing them with light and energy. The further you progress in your studies and the more you expand your imagination, the further you will unlock the mysteries behind the letters and their many beautiful postures.

Body

Poses:

Warrior II Pose

Reverse Warrior

Extended Side Angle Pose

Extended Triangle Pose and Variation

Warrior II Pose

Create the kavana (*intention*):

You are a channel connecting the energy of your soul in all directions. This powerful pose improves strength, stability, and concentration as it stretches the legs, groins, and chest.

Directions into the pose:

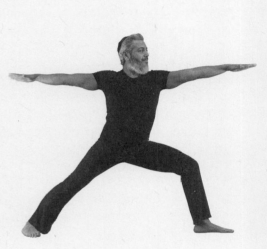

1. Step your feet three to four feet apart. Point your front foot forward and turn your back foot forty-five degrees toward the front of the mat.

2. Root down into the Earth.

3. Extend your arms from the heart, parallel to the ground.

4. Inhale and lift from your pelvic floor.

5. Feel energy spreading throughout your muscles, and open your shoulder blades wide.

6. Exhale, and bend your front knee over your ankle so the shin is perpendicular to the floor.

7. Energize your back leg and press the outer side of your foot firmly to the ground.

8. Lengthen the crown of your head above your lengthened spine.

9. Turn your gaze toward your fingers.

10. Imagine your soul spreading its energy from your body into the world.

11. Feel the space between your shoulder blades.

12. Take a few breaths and bring awareness to the lengthening of your torso upward and your arms to the sides, while your legs ground toward the Earth.

13. Inhale and release the pose.

14. Exhale and repeat on the other side.

Health and benefits:

- Improves breathing and increases stamina
- Releases tension in your neck and shoulders
- Tones and stretches the legs, ankles, arms, and abdomen
- Expands the chest and the lungs

Reverse Warrior

Create the kavana *(intention):*

Visualize drawing heaven into your heart as you stretch your arm into the sky. The pose requires stability and focus as you stretch the legs, heart, and arm.

Directions into the pose:

1. Start in Warrior II with the left foot forward, and bring the right hand down to rest softly on the back of your right leg.

2. Inhale, open your left palm to the sky, and reach your arm up above your head.

3. Keep your legs strong and rooted into the Earth.

4. To go further in the pose, bring your right hand to your heart, and while extending your whole upper body, bring the awareness of your breath into your heart and hand.

5. Return to Warrior II and repeat on the other side.

Health and benefits:

- Stretches the legs, hips, sides of torso, and waist

- Improves flexibility of the spine, ankles, inner thighs, and chest

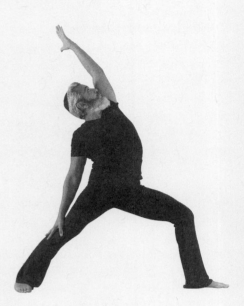

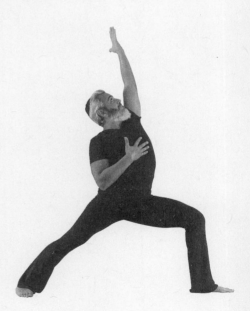

Extended Side Angle Pose

Create the kavana (*intention*):

Envision your heart filled with light, extending out and illuminating your body.

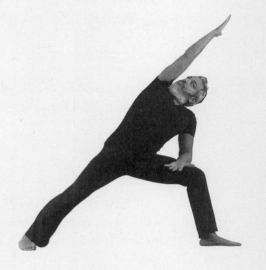

Directions into the pose:

1. Begin in Warrior II with the left leg forward.

2. Asymmetrically open your hips, aligning your torso over hips.

3. Extend your torso toward your left thigh.

4. Rest your arm on your thigh, tailbone rooted down toward the Earth.

5. Extend your other arm toward the sky.

6. Lift from your heart.

7. Lengthen the entire right side of your body over your thigh while rotating your chest up to the ceiling.

8. Turn your head toward your extended arm.

9. Release your left shoulder away from your ear.

10. Breathe in and out, creating space and length along both sides of your torso.

11. Push both heels strongly into the ground and reach up with your right hand as you come back up.

12. Repeat on the other side.

Health and benefits:

- Creates flexibility in the hip joints
- Improves balance and lengthens the spine
- Tones the abdomen
- Opens the chest and shoulders
- Strengthens the legs, knees, thighs, and ankles

Extended Triangle Pose and Variation

Create the kavana (*intention*):

See your heart as a window shining light into heaven and Earth. This deep pose stretches the hamstrings, groins, and hips while opening the chest and shoulders.

Directions into the pose:

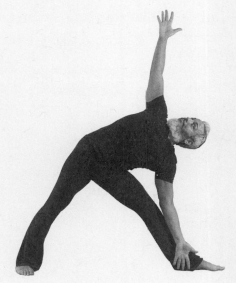

1. Step your feet three to four feet apart. Turn your front foot forward and pivot your back foot forty-five degrees toward the front, aligning your front heel with your back arch.

2. Bring your arms to shoulder height, and activate the lateral muscles of your torso.

3. Keep your back foot in firm contact with the ground.

4. Lengthen your torso energetically. The imaginary line from your tailbone to the heart should be a straight line of energy.

5. Radiate from your heart.

6. Imagine that your fingers reaching for the sky are shining like rays from your heart, receiving energy, and that your fingers touching the Earth are planting these rays from your heart as a piece of heaven, so they grow through you and within.

7. To go deeper into the pose, press down into your inner front leg, and extend the opposite arm over your head, keeping some space between your shoulders and ears.

8. Take the time to breathe deeply into the space you are creating.

9. Release the pose and repeat on the other side.

Health and benefits:

- Opens the heart chakra (energy field), which invites joy to fill the body

- Tones the spine and opens the hips

- Stimulates the abdominal organs while strengthening your legs and ankles

- Improves circulation and breathing

- Relieves stress

CHAPTER 2

BEIT: Home

Pose: Crescent Moon

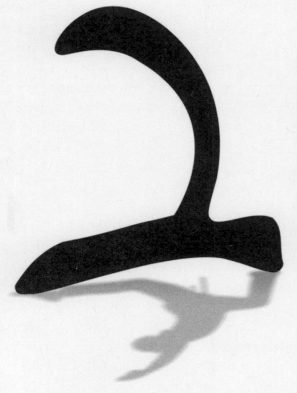

Your body is the home for your soul to find expression in thoughts, feelings, and actions.

The *Beit* corresponds to the English letter *B* and has a numerical value of 2.

Soul

Beit: Baniti, Yatsarti, Tikanti. "The home is founded on building, shaping, and healing."

—Akivah

Several years ago, my wife, Karen, and I decided that it was time to do renovations on our home. While Karen chose Mexican tiles for the floors and carefully arranged the furniture to give the feeling of openness, I had fun airbrushing a magnificent blue sky onto the ceiling, with clouds shaped like Hebrew letters! It is as though Karen had made the Earth, and I created heaven.

The sky with Hebrew letters on our ceiling is mesmerizing. One can be sitting on the couch and gaze upward at the letters and literally enter into a deep meditation. When we look out the windows at night, the shapes of the letters are reflected in the windows, resembling clouds and appearing as though the sacred shapes have flowed into our home from the outside.

This reminds me of the ancient story that says when the Creator was about to form a home in the world, the sacred letters hovered over him, with each one coming forward and expressing its desire to be the force behind this creation. Each letter approached the Creator separately to present its qualities. When the *Beit* came before the Creator, it simply said, "Let the world be created through me because I will bless this home." The Creator smiled and created the world with the sacred shape *Beit*.[1]

The *Beit* is physically shaped in a way that connects us to heaven and Earth. While it has an extended vertical "leg" to the Earth, it also has a lengthened horizontal "spine" that opens the heart. *Beit* has a value of two, and symbolizes pairs, unions, opposites and plurality, and characteristics of the Earth. The *Beit* also hints to the body and soul, you and me, we and the world, us and the Creator, yin and yang, right and left, and positive and negative. Some would even agree it is the unification of opposites.

The sages say that the Creator desired to build a home in the lowest of all worlds. The Creator's desire was motivated by the sacred shape of *Beit*, calling Earth a home, *bayit*, another way of pronouncing *Beit*. Before creation, there was only the Creator. It was he alone that existed. For millions of years, he made "vessels" and drew light into them. Each time, the vessels broke and shattered because the light was too powerful.

The Creator then began to envision our world, and drew deeply into his light, mixing it with compassion, causing the powerful light to become warm and tolerable. He then began to shade the light with his personality. Finally, there was hope and a glimpse of beauty that had been hidden was now awakened from within.

On the first day of creation, he imbued the potential life with his quality of kindness, and finally, a vessel strong enough to hold light was formed.

On the second day, the Creator breathed deeply from his essence and drew from his breath the skies and waters. In Genesis (chapter 1) it is written that in the beginning of creation, "*ruach* (the 'divine breath') hovered over the face of the waters." Oxygen came from heaven and entered the oceans, rivers, lakes, and all the other bodies of water. The sky then embraced his soul while the Earth took from his body. He made himself present through *ruach*—the divine breath that caused everything to come into existence and grow. He painted the ocean blue so the color of the sky would remind us that the waters are a reflection of heaven.

On the third day, the Creator added beauty to his creation by covering the ground with tones of brown and planting beautiful trees with various shades of green. He composed the sounds of nature as a symphony of Mother Earth. The sun, moon, and stars were made out of the Creator's external light and placed in the firmaments so they would provide light on Earth.

On the fourth day, the Creator made the stars and heavenly bodies. The movement of these help humans track time. Two great heavenly bodies were made in relation to the Earth. The first is the sun, which is the primary source of light, and the second is the moon, which reflects the light of the sun. The movement of these bodies distinguish day from night. This work was also declared by the Creator to be good. This creative work took one day.

On the fifth day, the Creator made the fish and other creatures of the oceans and lakes, and the birds that fly in the sky. All were made on the same day to tell us to search for the hidden secrets beneath the waters of life and that to be led by the freedom to become spiritual beings in human existence is to fly like birds toward heaven.

On the eve of the sixth day of creation, the animals were created. Then, at sunset, the Creator announced his plan to create humans in order to make a home on Earth. The sages say that the angels were surprised, and complained, "Here we are elevated and united with unlimited love and brotherhood. We serve you day and night. We have no conflict or jealousy among us. Why create humans to make your home if they are incomplete? Let us build your home!"

The Creator answered, "Earth is empty of light, and you can only live in light. I now imagined something different than light. I saw darkness in all its shades. Angels are made of light, and like the fish that can only survive in water, they can only survive as long as they are in light. Because humans can also live outside the light, they can make me a home on Earth."[2]

A home cannot be completely spiritual, as our physicality will never find its place of comfort. Moreover, if a home is only physical, then the spirit will never find expression.

The Letter

The letter *Beit* teaches us that a home is a space where we can nurture both our body and our soul in a way that makes us feel right at home.

In such an environment, where self-expression is at it ease, the space becomes your blessing. Your home reflects who you are. It is where the heart can open widely and deeply to express its emotions without reservations.

Without saying a word, your home can reveal what you do, how you live, and what you believe in. A home is your sacred space where your heart can fully reveal itself. It is where you can laugh, scream, and dance without holding back. It is the place of trust, confidence, warmth, and affection, where you can remove the masks that disguise your true self and be naked in the world.

The people of the world can often only see each other's outer layers. This happens because we create a veil of protection around us stemming from our worries and fears, and so we can avoid situations and people in our lives. The challenges we deal with daily at work or in our social circles teach us how to be strong in character. The aura we cultivate in our home, as our real self, can offer an immense life full of beauty and happiness, and lead to great character. To live in such a home, space must be made for your body and soul to be nourished. The home is also the home of the body and soul.

Whatever you may be experiencing in your body and soul will be felt in your actual home. Your home is your support system that holds you during your trials and challenges, and helps you grow into your desires. When you live in such a home, then the soul finds harmony and a rhythm of movement within the body.

Homes are certainly not perfect. Sometimes what appears on the outside is not necessarily a reflection of what's on the inside. But the opposite is also true. What we are on the inside reflects on the outside—even perception can be projection.

We have a choice to make. We can either see all the blessings in our lives, or we can focus on what's wrong and missing in our lives. The choices we make will affect the spirit of the home.

How do you make the world into a meaningful home? You begin with yourself, a personal home for your soul. You nourish your body and soul. You care for your mind, heart, and physical health. The *Beit* is a reminder to see the body as a temple, the carrier of the light of your soul. Your soul illuminates your body and home even when the light feels dim. Your soul inspires you to blossom into your best character. If a self-portrait or an autobiography were made of you, your home would most certainly be a starting point.

Our dream is to live our best life, to be happy and at peace, and to reach our dreams and goals. The soul may come and go into the world whether it is before or after your lifetime. Your body, however, will only materialize once as it has connected to your soul. In another lifetime, your soul may reemerge in a different form, such as a beautiful flower that will bring pleasure through its fragrance or a bird that will fly high into the sky. But for now, the only connection you need to consider is that of your actual body and the soul with which you have been blessed. Together they can ignite sparks on an Earth that sometimes feels dark.

If you open your heart to bringing more good into the world, the body becomes a sacred vessel where compassion, talent, passion, and skills become tools to make the world a beautiful home.

Breath: Energetic Shape and Intention

The kavanas *of the* Beit *are feelings of comfort in your body, sacredness in yourself, openness in your heart, and warmth in your life.* Beit *represents love, happiness, awareness of your blessings, and connection to Earth.*

The inhale of the letter is on the expansion of the heart as you lengthen your spine and reach your arms toward the sky. The exhale is the melting of the hips as you settle your body into the Earth while lengthening your back with your inner legs drawing unity into the midline of your body.

There are a few variations of the *Beit* we can assume: the Crescent Moon and its variations, including the Crescent Moon Low Lunge, Crescent Moon Lunge Variation, and Crescent Moon High Lunge.

When practiced with a feeling of comfort and satisfaction in the body and by opening the heart, the *Beit* becomes your reminder that your body is your temple and your heart is a sacred altar.

When shaping the body into the *Beit*, such as in the Crescent Moon Low Lunge, the extended back leg becomes a foundation to root yourself downward into the Earth and to hold as your body's home. The body is your temple. As you open your heart, you can imagine offering good feelings out to the universe.

In Crescent Moon High Lunge, as in a variation of Warrior I, the extended leg lifted from the Earth symbolizes an elevation of the body as you establish yourself downward to allow the emotions to rise higher from the heart. The inhale is the lengthening of the spine as you open your heart. The exhale is the rooting of the front foot and the pressing down of the mound of the back foot.

From the groundedness of the *Beit* comes your ability to soften emotions as you relax the hips and begin to open the heart to shine. The shape of the *Beit* is a reminder to open your heart while remaining connected to the Earth. According to Kabalah, the world is constructed according to the shape of the *Beit*.

The design of the *Beit* consists of three parts, which point to the directions east, south, and west. The arms extended upward and back represent the east. The spine and open heart represent the south, and the extended leg below it, the west. The open space represents the north and is formed between our extended arms and feet.

The *Beit* teaches the movement of the sun in our heart. For example, in the north the winter sun rises in the southeast and sets in the southwest. In the summer, the sun rises in the northeast and then sets in the northwest. A wonderful practice would be to bring awareness of the energy stemming from your heart. According to the sages, practicing yoga facing the south guides the sun's light into the different parts of your body.

You can also envision yourself as a crescent moon. If the universe is the sun, then we are the moon, a reflection of a higher light similar to the exchange of light between the sun and the moon. When in the *Beit* posture, by opening the heart while stretching the arms upward and evenly toward the back, we can see the shape of the moon being formed from the spine and arms. In the pose, feel your heart full of sun shining light.

Body

Poses:

Crescent Moon Low Lunge

Crescent Moon Lunge Variation

Crescent Moon High Lunge

Crescent Moon Low Lunge

Create the kavana (*intention*):

You are a habitation for your soul, a sacred space that carries light. The Crescent Moon Low Lunge is an important pose in yoga and is part of the traditional yoga warm-up sequences—called Salutations—because it warms up the body and uses all the muscles. By lengthening and enforcing your lower and upper body, you bring more balance and stability for opening the heart.

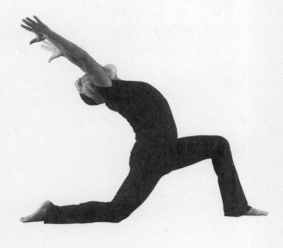

Directions into the pose:

1. Step forward and bring your left foot flat on the ground in front of your body in a runner's lunge position, using the forward movement to lift and open your heart. Place your hands on your front leg.

2. Square your hips.

3. Root into the Earth from your front leg through the four corners of your foot.

4. Bring your right knee down on the Earth and melt your hips forward.

5. Look straight ahead and sense yourself balancing.

6. Lift the energy of your body from your pubic bone into your heart.

7. Lengthen from the sides.

8. On an inhale, stretch your arms up and back over your head, allowing your upper body to follow. Keep your shoulder blades rooted to support the opening of your heart.

9. As you exhale, sink deeper into your groin area.

10. Come into Downward Dog, and repeat the pose on the other side.

Health and benefits:

- Opens the heart and back

- Opens the groin, which prepares the body for deeper backbends

- Encourages all the muscles of the body to work as one unit

- Creates a tremendous sense of balance and concentration, which will help promote a greater sense of inner peace

Crescent Moon Lunge Variation

Create the kavana (*intention*):

Envision yourself drawing deeper into your body as you allow your heart to explore the space you create in your body. This variation of Crescent Moon is a way of creating a space in your body that will grow its light into the space surrounding you.

Directions into the pose:

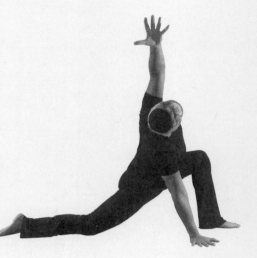

1. Begin in Crescent Moon Low Pose with the left leg forward.

2. Lean to the right. Place your right fingertips or palm on the floor.

3. Turn your bottom ribs toward the sky and broaden your collarbones. Lengthen your spine.

4. Stretch your left arm to the sky, creating a moon shape.

5. Keep your lower body rooted and feel the openness and space you are creating in your upper body.

6. After a few breaths, place your hands at your heart and move into Downward Dog for the transition.

7. Repeat on the other side.

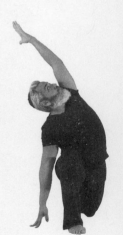

Health and benefits:

- Opens the upper body
- Softens the spine
- Expands the lungs
- Creates a deeper connection with the breathing process
- Promotes stability and groundedness

Crescent Moon High Lunge

Create the kavana *(intention):*

Envision your body, home of your soul, being elevated to higher realms ready to shine more light. The *Beit* in the High Lunge refers to the spiritual warrior within who transforms darkness into light. The difference between Crescent Moon High Lunge and Crescent Moon Low Lunge is that the former is done with the knee off the ground.

Directions into the pose:

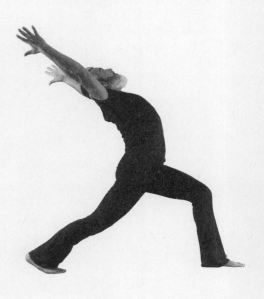

1. From the Crescent Moon Low Lunge, bring your hands to your heart, tuck in the toes of your back foot, and lift your knee away from the earth.

2. Press into your front foot, especially the heel mound.

3. Root the tailbone down and sink deeper.

4. Lift your arms parallel to each other and reach up through the fingertips toward the sky.

5. Extend from your hips all the way to your fingertips, allowing your heart to open. Root down your shoulder blades and soften your ribs, keeping your navel in.

6. Breathe into the beautiful shining light within you.

7. Repeat on the other side.

Health and benefits:

- Stretches the legs, groin, and hip flexors
- Opens the chest, heart, front torso, and shoulders
- Strengthens the thighs, buttocks, and hips
- Develops balance and stability

CHAPTER 3

GIMEL: Awareness in Kindness
Pose: Intense Side Stretch Pose

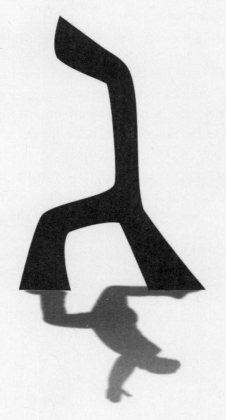

Kindness is the channel that unites us all into one body and soul.

The *Gimel* corresponds to the English letters G and J and has a numerical value of 3.

Soul

Gimel: Gamalti Yachad Me'Chasdim Le'dalim. "Connecting is drawing kindness into a receiver."

—Akivah

A story is told of a little fish who learned about water for the first time. He swam desperately from pond, to river, and then to the ocean, searching for water. One day a wise old fish noticed the wandering little fish searching for something. He stopped him and helped him realize that he had actually been swimming in water all his life, and he just needed to become aware of it. "It's right here in front of you, and all around you," he said. The little fish became enlightened, and began his journey back home with the awareness that he has always been surrounded by that which he was searching for. It was always right in front of him and surrounded him at all times.

This story teaches us two lessons: one of awareness, and the other, how to engage awareness by simple acts of kindness, which is the meaning of *Gimel*.

Awareness is similar to understanding the divine breath and the air, or ether, that surrounds and fills all of existence. Since creation, divine breath has been constantly creating and recreating everything in the universe out of nothingness. We may not see it, but it is everywhere and affects everything in our lives. It's a grid of universal awareness, folding and unfolding upon itself. Personal awareness, once realized, shapes our perception and reaction to situations. Like our breath, we can learn to master awareness by influencing it to be short and shallow, or long, deep, and meaningful. We will start to breathe differently, more calmly and smoothly, depending on how we react in a moment of awareness. We can become more settled, focused, and present in the moment.

The Letter

Gimel, pronounced "gamol," means to draw inward and reach awareness. Awareness is not something unreachable or limited to a select few. Rather, it is something to cultivate from within. It is nothing more than being present in our body, mind, and heart. Achieving vibrations of a higher realm, or blissful state, is important to us, and awareness within connects us deeper to our heart. Drawing inward is not an activity of the mind, but the development of a feeling heart that understands connection. The key is to feel.

Kabalah explains that the waters of the oceans, rivers, and lakes symbolize the hidden world of our inner and higher self where all the deep secrets of life are concealed. The Earth body is the revealed world where all things can become known. The fish (*nunei yama* or "creatures of the waters") represent the soul gathered into the source of life where it bathes in the infinite light. Before we descended on Earth, our soul lived within the infinite light. The wise fish is the *Tzadik*, an old soul who acts as our teacher and guru, and often our inner voice guiding us onto the path of our life's destiny. We become lost in our search for truth in the great waters that often flood our vision when we have disconnected or forgotten to tune in. The old fish is the voice within, reminding us to open our eyes wider in order to see deep into ourself, to find silence and even sense, or feel, our connection to the universe and others.

Such an awareness assumes that we are rooted in a higher vibration that clearly sees the big picture, the greatest our soul can envision, before us. Our experience in a moment of enlightenment, the feeling of absolute awareness, begins to grow deeply within our body and nourishes this spark of awareness. It begins pushing into every part of us, all the way down to our DNA.

The *Gimel* teaches us to be more present—physically, mentally, and emotionally—when engaged in an action that brings us into contact with another person. For example, we can do a favor for someone without feeling or thought, and become agitated. Or, we can be engaged fully and present in our involvement with others, happy to lend a helping hand. Our actions are something we can control, similar to controlling a dimmer switch to augment or decrease the light's intensity. Sometimes it is about adding more light into a space to create clarity. Other times we need to lower the light in order to get a better sense of our surroundings and achieve more understanding without our two physical eyes. We need all three eyes to become fully aware! To be aware, we also need to search inward to find the inner light that is sometimes hidden from our pain and suffering. The ray of light will reveal truth once the gem in the rough—our soul—becomes revealed.

Like the fish in the water unaware of his surroundings, we are, and have always been, surrounded by light. It is even within us. We are made from the light. In the same way that the fish can only survive in water, we can only exist in the eternal light. The difference is how in tune we become with the light in our life, as we control the dimmer switch of our soul. So, the first lesson of the *Gimel* is to be engaged with yourself in order to be open to more awareness.

Another lesson of the story of the fish is about engaging our awareness through the meaning of *Gimel*, which is kindness. Kindness is beneficial for both our physical and our emotional well-being. Research confirms that any act of kindness stimulates the vagus nerve, which warms the heart area and stimulates the brain's emotional center by releasing dopamine, the hormone that helps us feel positive emotions and find happiness. Kindness reduces stress, depression, and nervousness.[3] It helps us create bonds with others—even total strangers.

The wise old fish teaches us that it is important to recognize the lost fish that we may come across, and to take a moment to help a wanderer find his or her way. The wise old fish is our infinite soul that has existed in many lives and bodies. It's telling us to look within and see our true reality, a prism of possibilities. There are only possibilities to be seen.

We can see from our two physical eyes and process this information into our brain, which then draws itself into our heart using the pineal gland to create feelings, which can then be translated into actions. But when we see from the soul, we are looking beyond the surfaces, layers, and physical bodies. The windows in the black holes of our eyes connect us to the light of the soul shining inside. Have you ever stared into the eyes of another for a long period of time? It can be an emotional shared moment.

When we create a bond, we are joining our common light to form a more powerful light in union. The more light there is, the more awareness can be experienced. When we see from the soul, everything is clearer and moves into harmony. Until we have made the effort to see life around us from a deeper perspective, we will remain as a little fish swimming into the ocean of life, searching for answers with no real direction or understanding. The more we become attuned to the voice of our soul within our heart, the more we see our days on Earth as great opportunities to connect with other souls—to facilitate bringing out the wise old fish in each of us.

We do not have to wait for another person's direction to do an act of kindness. We need to search for these moments inside ourselves first by creating space and time. The heart energy develops the desire to simply want to help others. We can then grow out of our occupation with ourselves to share our gifts of personality, skills, and talents with one another.

We must be grateful that we can both give and receive regardless of our roles in society. To be able to give and receive is a great blessing that generates energy for all. The *Gimel* serves as a great lesson that each act of generosity, kindness, compassion, and understanding is the binding force that holds the world together by bringing us closer to the source of love. Always know that the person you reach out to is equally important. The receiver is our partner in life. The giver must remember that if they have something to give, it is a gift from a higher realm or vibration and yet a privilege that can be taken away at any time. The giver may sense a mission or purpose with someone in an act of kindness. The receiver is a vehicle that completes the connection of two souls through the expression of gratitude. Whether we are the receiver or giver, when there is awareness to our thoughts, words, and actions, we become a conduit for translating the higher light vibration into energy that warms the heart with love, benevolence, compassion, understanding, beauty, and so much more.

Breath: Energetic Shape and Intention

The kavanas of the Gimel are feelings of love, compassion, gratitude, understanding, softness in your heart, warmth in your body, and awareness of being rooted, grounded, and connected to all beings, animals, and things of the Earth.

One way of doing the *Gimel* is to let your hands flow together with clasped fingers and stretch up and back, stretching the arms to the sky as the heart rises from the chest out to the universe. Then exhale, rooting down from the front foot as you even the hips. Connect the back foot to the Earth, lengthen the leg, and draw energy into the pelvis, heart, and mind.

The *Gimel* can be shaped according to the Intense Side Stretch Pose as well as its variations. Also, the *Gimel* resembles the Bridge Pose with one leg extended.

The intention of the *Gimel* is to acquire feelings of love and gratitude for yourself and others. It reminds us that we are conduits for carrying kindness in all its forms, whether as receivers or as givers. Caring for ourselves begins the path toward kindness for others. The more we honor life, the further will it benefit our surroundings. Kindness is conveyed in the image of the letter *Gimel*. *The Talmud* tells us that the shape of the letter resembles a person wishing to perform kindness.

In the *Gimel,* the feet are pressed to the ground to show stability while the hands are held back either on the hips, clasped behind to open the heart, or toward the sky, reaching for a greater awareness as the head faces forward, focused on connecting to light. In all variations, the heart is open and receptive to feelings that trigger kindness.

The *Gimel* in the Intense Side Stretch Pose is shaped by standing with your legs apart and hips even. As you extend your arm to the sky, inhale and imagine connecting through the tips of your fingers to the source of light. When folding over your front leg, exhale, and tap into the energy of opening your heart and extending your arm over your head. Think of reaching out to others with love, warmth, and sincerity. You can envision as though you are the *Gimel* extending toward the Earth and all its creations with the energy of the heart leading the way. We can live with the teaching of the *Gimel* by practicing loving-kindness and gratitude for all we have.

You may also lie flat on your back, as in the Bridge Pose with Leg Extended, with your arms by your sides, clasped under you, or over your head. Lift on an inhale one leg toward the sky and imagine having one foot rooted into heaven. Exhale, root your other foot into the Earth, keeping the heart inspired and lifted to draw energy into the body.

Body

Poses:

Intense Side Stretch Pose (Pyramid) with Arms Extended

Intense Side Stretch Pose Variations

Bridge Pose with Leg Extended

Intense Side Stretch Pose (Pyramid) with Arms Extended

Create the kavana (*intention*):

You are a body of kindness—a conduit for spreading light from your soul. Physically, the movement in Intense Side Stretch Pose consists of actions that require grounding, centering, and a deepening into the pose.

Directions into the pose:

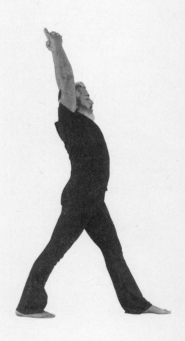

1. Come to standing with your feet together and arms by your sides, and think about yourself as a carrier of light. Breathe with awareness.

2. Root down into the Earth and notice your body weight flowing downward.

3. Tuck in your tailbone and draw in your abdomen.

4. Step your feet four feet apart and place your hands on your hips.

5. Turn your left foot forward and pivot your right foot so it points to the right corner of your mat.

6. Turn your hips, torso, and head toward the right so you are facing forward.

7. Inhale and lengthen your arms toward the sky.

8. Exhale, soften your shoulders, and energize your legs, lengthening the tailbone down and bringing the navel in.

9. Inhale, and open your heart to heaven.

10. To go further into the pose, exhale, bend your elbows, and bring your hands in prayer behind your head with fingers pointing downward.

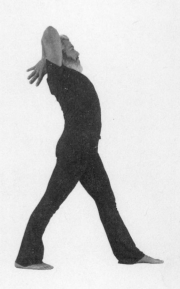

11. Settle into your sacred body.

12. Allow your spine to curve as you continue to feel the extension of the front of your body.

13. Breathe as you contemplate being an extension of goodness.

14. Repeat on the other side.

Health and benefits:

- Strengthens the legs
- Improves posture and balance
- Stretches the spine, shoulders, wrists, hips, and hamstrings
- Relaxes the brain

Intense Side Stretch Pose Variations

Create the kavana (*intention*):

You are the prayer of the heart, an inner voice that expresses the yearning of the light to shine.

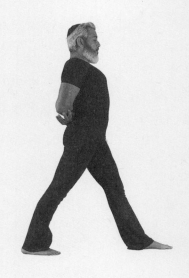

Directions into the pose:

1. Begin in Intense Side Stretch Pose.

2. Draw down from heel to ball, and point your tailbone toward the Earth.

3. Straighten your torso, open your arms sideways, rotate your shoulders in, and bring your hands into Reverse Prayer Pose.

4. Breathe with awareness as you look inside your soul.

5. Lift your spine as you open your heart more deeply.

6. Ground down equally through both legs.

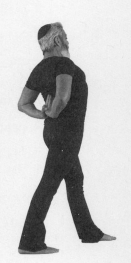

7. To take the pose further, release the prayer hands and move into lengthening your arms behind you with fingers clasped.

8. Inhale, and open toward the sky, leading from your heart. Exhale, and bend forward, bringing your heart over your front leg, releasing the spine.

9. Surrender to relax your neck, and allow your head to accept the pull of gravity.

10. Connect to the Earth, channeling energy from your fingers.

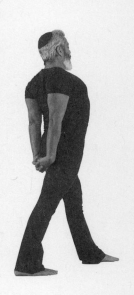

11. Draw your arms slightly up toward the sky, squeezing your shoulder blades into your back and toward one another.

12. Feel your chest opening, and with each breath, allow yourself to sink down as you bend from your hips, bringing your torso closer to the thigh of your front leg.

13. Bring lightness into your body; imagine the sky opening into your heart as it draws its light into the Earth.

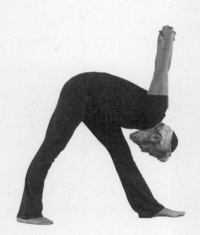

14. Envision the energy of the Earth rising into your legs, hips, torso, chest, heart, and mind as your legs stand strong, supporting your body.

15. Feel grounded and connected to the Earth, the source of physical life.

16. From your hips, bring yourself back up, arms by your sides, and standing at the front of your mat.

17. Repeat on the other side.

Health and benefits:

- Opens the hips

- Stretches the calves and hamstrings

- Supports the wrists, and increases mobility of the shoulders

- Massages the abdominal organs when the head rests on the knee

Bridge Pose with Leg Extended

Create the kavana *(intention):*

Envision lifting your entire life toward the sky and connecting with it.

Directions into the pose:

1. Lie flat on your back with your arms at your sides.

2. Connect to the energy underneath you.

3. Bend both knees, and place your feet flat on the floor directly below your knees, hip-width apart.

4. Scoop your tailbone under and lift your hips up; keep resting your shoulders on the Earth.

5. Breathe and lift your hips a little bit more.

6. Rest your head, neck, and shoulders on the Earth, softly relaxed.

7. Think about being a vehicle for sharing kindness.

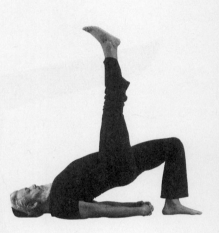

8. Keep your eyes focused directly above you on the sky or ceiling.

9. Do not move your head or neck from side to side.

10. Lift one leg and bring a flexed foot up toward the sky.

11. Keep your hips lifted, tailbone lengthened.

12. Lower your hips and repeat on the other side.

Health and benefits:

- Opens the chest and the abdominal wall

- Stimulates the thyroid and improves digestion

- Relieves mild depression

- Tones the buttocks and the thighs

- Stabilizes the lower back

- Creates a deeper connection with the breathing process

CHAPTER 4

DALET: Word

Pose: Warrior III

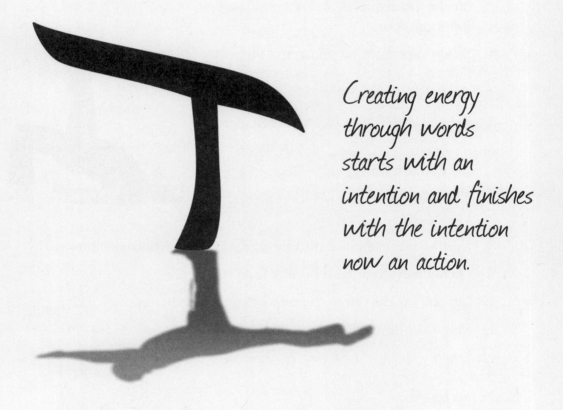

*Creating energy
through words
starts with an
intention and finishes
with the intention
now an action.*

The *Dalet* corresponds to the letter *D* and has a numerical value of 4.

Soul

Dalet: Devarai Le'Olam. "The sacred word is forever."

—Akivah

A student was being tested by his teachers in what they said would be improvised speech. They told him that they would not give him the text of the sermon until he was on the pulpit facing the congregation.

The time came, and the young aspirant went to the pulpit, where he found a folded slip of paper. When he opened it, to his surprise, it was completely blank. For the first few seconds, he turned the empty paper over and over again as he stood, uncertain how to react. He then looked into the eyes of his audience, took a deep breath, and began his speech: "Nothing on this side, and nothing on that side. In the beginning there was nothing, and out of this nothingness everything came to be."

Before anything existed, there was only the Creator.[4] It was he himself, and nothing else existed. He is *ein sof,* "the eternal light." The sages explain that he is the *ein sof* because his light that illuminates everything is no-thing. It is called "the light of nothing" because there is no-thing except for it. It is *ein* because nothing exists except for the Creator, *sof.* The light is everything because his light shines in each thing, revealed or concealed, independent of whether it is from Earth, animal, or human. The *ein sof,* light of nothing and in everything, is therefore revealed in all realities while simultaneously hidden in all concealment.

To make a world, the Creator envisioned making the no-thing into everything physical by piercing an empty space within the vast light of himself. He contracted and withdrew from his light by lowering and screening it until a void was carved out within the light itself. The mystics say that at this auspicious moment, the Creator began breathing deeply, and from his depth, started his long-awaited speech that would make out of nothing a something—the Earth.

The Letter

This was the Creator's most powerful speech that brought the world into existence through *dibur,* "powerful words," which is the meaning of the letter *Dalet.*

The sages explain that the speech given was in *Lashon Hakodesh,* the sacred tongue then only known by the Creator and the celestial beings. This ancient language is made up of the Hebrew letters, and by combining them into words, each thing was formed as the vibration of his voice penetrated the very fabric of heaven and Earth.

Mantra, a Sanskrit word, is the common term used in reference to words that instill depth and can bring about change within us. In Hebrew, a mantra is a *dibur*. Saying a mantra or *dibur* with awareness can fill the mind, heart, and body with positive transformation.

The Hebrew letters used by the Creator in forming words to make the world are sacred and contain great powers. When meaningful words are formed and repeated with intention, they become energetic channels that can have great influence.

When comparing the four kingdoms of the Earth—the inorganic, vegetative, animal, and human—Kabalah refers to humans as the *me'daber*, "man of words," because words are our greatest asset.

Words have an influence on our mood, situation, and perception of life. When words are positive, loving, and considerate, they can be illuminating, uplifting, motivating, and inspiring. When words are spoken from the heart-center where body meets soul, they enter into another heart and allow us to feel gratitude, love, compassion, happiness, joy, peace, and confidence. Such words purify the air surrounding us and bring more life and vitality into all who say, hear, or are affected by words.

Sometimes words are hard and painful, and make us feel sad and broken inside. The sages warn us that when one gossips, they hurt themselves, the person listening, and the one being talked about. Why is the one being spoken of affected by the gossip if they are not part of the conversation? Because words spoken with intention, whether positive or negative, have power over us and therefore even the third person, the subject, will be touched by the negative conversation.

To speak from the heart requires humility, another meaning of the letter *Dalet*. Humility is often associated with simplicity or poverty. To be humble does not mean to underestimate your true worth. Humility is the greatest sign of wisdom, and will certainly cause our words to be heard.

Moses was one of the greatest men who ever lived, and yet the Bible tells us that he was the most humble of all men. Although he stuttered when he spoke, still he is considered the greatest orator of ancient times. Humility is knowing that we are a nothing and yet a something here on Earth to serve the universe. It is being grateful for all you have and expressing this by being willing to share with others.

A humble person understands that they own nothing in this world. Everything they have was lent to them by the universe to help make their mission on Earth successful. The *Dalet* tells us that humility is seeing that there is a greater force that controls all forces of nature. We exist in this space to receive and give back what we have. Whether you are giving of yourself or receiving from another, both are important in filling the emptiness.

We can learn from the *Dalet* to develop this quality of humility as an empowerment to achieving great things in our life and to appreciate the magnificence of kindness as the binding force between us and others. When there is modesty, the heart becomes more motivated to reach out and share inspiration.

The sages compare a word to a body and its intention to its soul. The expression of both the body and the soul as one existence will come through a humble heart. Because the heart is the center of our existence, it is the most important organ that will influence what we say and how we will be heard. When the body is warmed from words spoken from the heart, our mind becomes warmed, and when this happens, our actions will also be affected. If the body of our words embraces the sincerity and inner depth of the soul, then higher life arises and will affect this very moment. The power of the heart is such that not only will the now be transformed in a more exalted way, but the moments and instances that will come right after will also feel the heart intention you create. For this reason, the sages advised their students to always repeat sacred words even while walking the streets of their city. This, they would say, will cleanse not only the surrounding air we breathe but also the air underneath us with each step we take upon the Earth with intention.[5] The Earth receives an aha moment each time we walk upon it with a positive intention expressed through words and feelings.

Creating energy through our words is a process that starts with a thought, *machshava*, and finishes with an action, *ma'aseh*. The words, *dibur*, we use to express the thought are the bridge between intention and experience. We can begin to energize our words by clearing our mind through breathing with awareness and meditation. Awareness of our breath can be as simple as expanding and contracting more deeply, or feeling and listening to our breath. Meditation can be sitting comfortably in stillness in a quiet space, or walking in nature and calming the raging mind and nervous system. An intention can then be cultivated in this space we make internally, and, depending upon the degree of awareness we reach, certain feelings will be born from the heart.

Repeating a *dibur* several times becomes an inner movement that vibrates in the body and in the heart. This physical vibration is the act of cultivating the word internally as its energy spreads into every part of our body and levels of consciousness.

A positive word will be heard in the body and echo into every limb, organ, bone, cell, and molecule. When the intention of the word meditated on is finally settled within as a seed planted into the Earth, positive reactions will emerge from the soil of our heart. At the moment the body captures the essence of a special word grown from the heart, it comes closer to the soul and new intelligence starts to rise from the body. The self takes on a higher embrace of life by now seeing itself as a temple, the heart as an altar, the mind as the sky, and the breath as a divine offering.

Breath: Energetic Shape and Intention

The kavanas of the Dalet are feelings of stability, focus, harmony, freedom, awareness of the energy surrounding you, humility, and depth.

The *Dalet's* main pose is Warrior III and requires stability, strength, focus, and lightness. The inhale is at the lifting of the body above the standing leg. The exhale is on the shining through your standing leg downward into the Earth. The inhale is also the opening of the heart upward and extension of the arms radiating with light. The exhale is the expanding forward of the sternum and focusing, as you draw toward the center and maintain an elevation of the body with awareness of the energy surrounding you.

The *Dalet* consists of two lines, one vertical and the other horizontal. The top line symbolizes your mind connecting to your heart as the body is lifted. The horizontal line represents the drawing of this balanced energy into the Earth. The more grounded you are into the four corners of your supporting foot, the more balanced you will be as you rise higher. The sages say that the space between the vertical and horizontal lines is open for the heart to find its full expression with the support of the mind and body. Your heart is also the contact between the body and the soul rooted in the same light. The body, and its qualities in thought, feelings, and actions, is the platform for the soul to be revealed. The more we cultivate ourselves spiritually as we do physically, we find harmony that works internally as well as externally. The heart is the navigator that brings the body closer to the soul. With the heart, we can share deep feelings through meaningful words that will enter another heart and express what is in our heart's essence.

The Warrior III, the main pose of the *Dalet*, is a balancing pose, which creates stability throughout the body by rooting your supporting leg into the Earth, while shining from your heart into the extension of your arms and lifted leg.

When doing the *Dalet*, you will notice that to rise higher, you need to be grounded. The shape of the pose makes you aware of the energy underneath as you root the foot down to the Earth and lift the body. By harnessing the energy in your center, you bring awareness to the energy surrounding your body, lifting and connecting to the energy above you.

In Warrior III, you can envision the body grounded and the heart blossoming as you fly high into a feeling of liberation. The freedom of the *Dalet* will depend upon how grounded you are on the supporting leg. The more you are rooted, the more you can feel elevated in spirit and in heart. The *Dalet* teaches how, in one posture and on one leg, we can lift an entire world and find our expression.

When you extend your arms out to the sides or to the front, envision that you are freeing yourself from any holding back as you fly into the energetic space around you. By remaining balanced and strong, you can draw energy into the heart, the main organ for tasting freedom.

Balancing in Warrior III is challenging. Cultivating focus and balance necessitates humility. Extending ourselves while doing this pose, or when reaching to another person, can make us feel as though we are falling forward. The sages say each imbalance is for a greater steadiness and therefore is never a fall but an opportunity to grow stronger and more rooted.

Alternatively, when you sit on the Earth, as in the Staff Pose, you prepare the body for poses that are deeper. This improves your concentration, while enhancing the essential keys for alignment in your body. As you connect to the Earth, you can envision your upper body, on an inhale, lifting your heart and mind into one line of energy and drawing from underneath you, on an exhale, to what is above you.

The physical benefits of the Staff Pose also touch us spiritually. When the upper part of the body is strong, the heart can open wider and allow more expression of the inner self.

Light is symbolic of the spine extending from the navel and connecting to the heart, through the pubic bone, sternum, and crown of the head. The extended legs of the Staff Pose represent the physical realm where we cultivate stability through our body actions.

The sages recount that the *Dalet* gave life to the four forms of existence: inorganic, vegetable, animal, and human. By connecting to the *Dalet*, whether in the Warrior III or Staff Pose, we also unite with these four realms of consciousness and bring more life to our inner four elements of Earth (body, action, experience), fire (heart, feelings, intention), water (mind, stillness, flow), and air (breath, awareness, essence).

Body

Poses:

Warrior III Pose

Staff Pose

Warrior III Pose

Create the kavana (*intention*):

Envision your body as a beam of light being lifted and expressing radiant light. Focus on your standing foot as a point of balance, and feel your weight equally distributed among the heel, the base of the big toe, and the base of the little toe.

Directions into the pose:

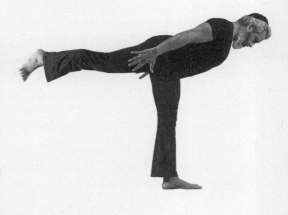

1. As you prepare for the pose in Mountain Pose, bring your palms together to your heart. Breathe steadily.

2. Inhale, shift all your weight into your supporting leg, and root down on all four corners of the standing foot. Exhale, and lift your leg up behind you as you fold your torso forward.

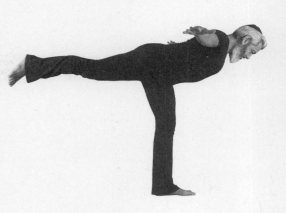

3. Stretch your arms backward, beside your hips.

4. Align your hips by internally rotating the upper thighs.

5. Inhale, and lengthen your spine from your tailbone to the crown of your head.

6. Exhale, and lengthen your tailbone toward your back heel.

7. Focus on one spot on the floor in front of you.

8. To feel the sensation of your heart radiating, stretch your arms out to the sides.

9. Envision your mind clearing. Breathe softly, and feel that you are radiating with energy from the heart to the feet and hands.

10. Visualize your body in a straight line from your heels to your fingertips. Your chest and leg are parallel to the floor, creating a feeling of stillness above the Earth.

11. If you feel shaky, bend your standing leg slightly and press deeply into the Earth.

12. Hold for five breaths.

13. Repeat on the other side.

Health and benefits:

- Improves balance, and physical, mental, and psychological power
- Stretches the entire length of the spine
- Increases circulation throughout the body
- Strengthens the capacity of the lungs
- Improves posture

Staff Pose

Create the kavana *(intention):*

Imagine your spine as a line of light firmly rooted in the Earth, extending vertically from the core to the crown of your head. Although seated Staff Pose may seem simple, it is the foundation to all seated postures, and it builds strength in the upper back, abdomen, and chest while requiring mental focus.

Directions into the pose:

1. Sit on the floor and extend your legs forward.

2. If you are experiencing tight hamstrings, lift the pelvis by sitting on a blanket or a bolster.

3. Plant your hands next to your hips.

4. Firm the thighs and press them down into the Earth, connecting to the energy underneath you.

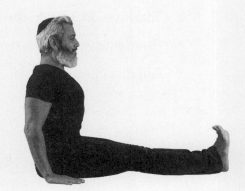

5. Slightly rotate your thighs toward each other by drawing the inner groins toward the sacrum.

6. Flex your feet and press out through your heels.

7. Keep your big toes together and imagine pressing your feet against a wall.

8. Inhale, root your hands down, and lengthen through the crown of your head, connecting to the energy above you.

9. Exhale, and gaze straight ahead, toward the horizon, as you connect to the Earth underneath you.

10. Visualize the energy of light moving upward from the pubis to the chest and sternum, and then streaming down the back from the shoulders to the tailbone.

11. Draw your shoulders back and feel your collarbones broadening.

12. Sit tall and ground your sitting bones into the Earth as you soften your front ribs.

13. Embrace the energy light and shine.

Health and benefits:

- Strengthens and lengthens the spine, upper back, shoulders, abdomen, and chest

- Stretches the shoulders and chest

- Benefits posture and alignment

- Improves focus, calms the mind, and brings relaxation to the entire body

CHAPTER 5

HEIH: Breath

Pose: One-Legged Extension

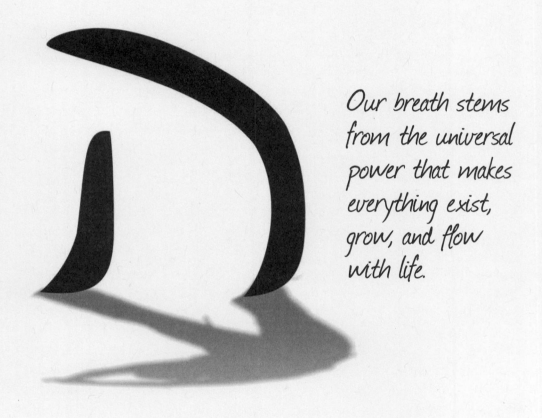

Our breath stems from the universal power that makes everything exist, grow, and flow with life.

The *Heih* corresponds to the English letter *H* and has a numerical value of 5.

Soul

Heih: Ha'Shamayim VeHa'retz Be' Heih'Baram. "Heaven and Earth were created through *Heih* (breath)."

—Akivah

As a child, I played a game with my friends at the pool where we would count the seconds and see who could hold his breath longer underwater. The last one that would emerge was the winner. This game was a lot of fun as we breathed with freedom and innocence, cutting off our own breath. Little did we know that as adults, breathing with control would be the most important step in dealing with life's many challenges.

We were too young then to realize that this game had to do with the soul. Children are not usually taught to breathe with awareness or that our breath comes from the soul. Our parents and teachers of life showed us how to have manners, eat properly, sleep at normal hours, use the toilet, read, write, and develop qualities. For some reason, no one thought that teaching children about breathing with consciousness was an important tool of life. Unless you grew up exposed to yoga, meditation, or breathing with awareness, it will be one of the things in life you learn on your own.

As we get older and as our innocence slowly begins to fade away, our breath thickens because of the challenges in our lives. We need to remember our inner child and find our first breath.

Life began with breath, the power of the letter *Heih*. Breath stems from the universal power that makes everything exist, grow, and move. We connect to the world by inhaling its air and exhaling our own breath back into it. No matter who you are, your breath is important for yourself and for the world around you.

Prior to your soul's descent, it met on high with the Creator to discuss its mission on Earth. All the wisdom necessary was given to you at that moment to fulfill your dreams and aspirations. As you were about to come into the world, the Creator tapped you below your nose and carved a medial cleft, signaling that you have been personally endowed with the Creator's breath.

Breath starts its first pulsations when we are in our mother's womb, surrounded by an ocean of breath. When we leave the womb, the first inhale we take is the initial contact our soul makes with our body, now separate from the mother. After a long, beautiful life, we ascend to heaven through an exhalation that brings our soul back to its maker.

From the moment we are born, breathing is automatic and natural. A healthy baby has the wisdom to breath effortlessly. For months, until it can finally move around and crawl, breathing is its main activity. Ever notice a baby while lying on its back? Its whole body naturally gets into the pulsation of expansion and contraction of its breath. When we get older, however, this natural breath slowly disappears, without ever realizing that our life is dependent upon it. Breath is so essential to life that without it, we could never survive, even for a few moments. Awareness of your breath can improve your daily habits, improve your posture, lead to clearer thoughts, and open you to awareness.

Awareness of your breath affects your body, heart, and mind, and will influence how you perceive and react to challenges in life. Whatever you are going through, the status of your breath will determine how you experience your situations mentally, emotionally, and physically. If you are in pain or in a weakened state, your breath will be abnormal, weak, and short. If you are happy or joyful, your breath will be fuller and energetic. When you meditate, sit in stillness, or pray deeply from the heart, your breath will feel flowing, smooth, and calm. If you lose touch with your breath, your connection to your body weakens, and your soul's relevance begins to diminish. When this occurs, the heart feels hardened, similar to a tight muscle, and the breath becomes irregular, especially in difficult situations.

At times it is as though there is almost no more breath in you. You are unable to take deep or lengthened breaths. You thirst for fresh air as though you were drowning underwater in your challenges. Breathing deeply helps you reconnect to that childlike breath where your whole body moves with your breath. Breathing with awareness should feel natural, and it is; it's just that we can be so immersed in our daily challenges that we forget the freedom our breath can offer in difficult times. Noticing your breath is a good way to start letting go of your worries and anxieties and freeing yourself from limitations. You do not need to think in order to breathe. Instead, what is required is awareness of your presence right here and now, breathing life, growing from your soul.

The Letter

The sound of an exhale from your mouth is the sound one makes when pronouncing *Heih*, like "heihhhhh!"

Exhaling the sound of the *Heih* through your mouth brings calmness and relaxation. What we can perceive as we breathe in and out is an image of life expanding and contracting. We are always either taking in or giving out, and so the exhale is as important as the inhale. The sound of breath can be discerned when we close our sense of hearing to what is outside of us and focus on the sound of the inner movement of our breath.

Try this for a moment: Inhale through your nose, hear the "ssou" sound and exhale from your mouth. Notice the "heihhhh" sound. Repeat a few times. Listen to the *Heih* inside your breath. It is soft, smooth, and soothing. It is telling you that you are alive and have a soul.

Awareness of your breath as it deepens, expands, contracts, and embraces allows you to channel your energy more powerfully throughout your body. It is not just how you inhale but also how you exhale into every part of you, which affects your mood, nervous system, posture, and soul.

The Zohar, a principal work of Kabalah, explains that the right nostril provides life and vitality for the entire body, allowing the heart to pulsate, the blood to flow, and the lungs to expand, and is known as *hayin*, or "vitality." The left nostril, whose purpose is to stimulate intelligence of the body and of the soul, leads to expression, creativity, and deeper understanding (*da'at*) is called *hayin de'hayin*, "vitality of life." Both are important and serve the purpose of keeping us alive and sensitive to the energy within and surrounding us, without which we could not exist. The *hayin* and the *hayin de'hayin* are the channels that allow us to experience with our body, feel from our heart, think with our mind, and be from our soul. The difference, however, is in the way we perceive and use the energy we receive from the nostrils. The body is dependent upon food, water, movement, and many other things in order to live. The soul, however, requires nothing it does not already have. Because it came from nothing, it is nothing because we cannot touch, hear, or see it as we do with anything in our body or in this world. We can, however, experience the soul by breathing with awareness. This action is divine, and is directly connected with the Creator. When breathing deeply, we can feel this movement embracing us from inside, touching us everywhere in our body.

Now try this: Place both hands on your chest and breathe deeply from your nose. Inhale and exhale a few times. Deepen your breath as you take in and give out air. Do it with the consciousness that your breath is moving internally to your chest. Next, do this with your hands on your ribs and then on your belly, and repeat a few times. Breathe deeply into your body. Notice how your breath expands and grows in different parts of your body. The more you become aware of your breath as it grows in every part of you, the more you will connect to your soul, connect to the energy of your inner body, and come closer to the essential breath of creation that made all life possible.

The health of the soul is not something that we could come to know by appearance only. Nor is it something that we can, or should, come to occasionally. The soul is something we must nourish as much as we do the body. We can begin to know the soul by learning about our breath. When we breathe from the mouth, we reach into the heart as a pathway into the essence of the body. When we breathe from the nose, we glimpse into the infinite wisdom passing through the mind. Both lead to the soul. The body cannot exist without the soul giving it life. The soul could not shine without a body. The mind would not have expression if the soul did not constantly nourish it with light. The heart could not spread its warmth into the organs if the soul did not give its *neshimah*, or "breath." Bringing awareness to your breath means feeling the breath entering your body and listening to the soft sound of the air traveling throughout your body, and then slowly letting go of any tension, stiffness, and distraction. Let your thoughts pass by and focus on melting away strain while releasing blockages inside you.

Breath: Energetic Shape and Intention

The kavanas of the Heih are the soothing feeling of your breath as it comes into your body, the expansion and contraction of your heart, and the warming of your body. It is finding energy within the space between each breath that arouses, renews, rejuvenates, and inspires.

In Hebrew, the word for breath, *neshimah,* consists of the same letters as the word for the soul, *neshamah.* These words contain two ideas: *neshim heih* and *nesham hah*, meaning the "breath of the letter *Heih*" and the "soul of the letter *Heih*." While the breath of the letter *Heih* represents its physical quality and acts as your body's energy and physical expressions, the *hah* sound is the soul, your inner light, simplicity, and spirit yearning to shine.

Breathing with awareness heals the mind and body. By learning how to be conscious of your breath, you can improve your daily habits and adopt better posture and clearer thoughts. Breathing deeply helps you cope with stress and tension, and empowers you to focus on your inner self and discover new strengths you never knew you had. Awareness of the breath allows you to understand your life's patterns and how you ended up where you are today. Your breath emanates from your soul. In the practice of yoga, your awareness of your breath will be the glue that connects your physical movement to the flow of your soul.

With consciousness of breath, you will feel yourself opening your mind and body to fuel up with new energy. The soul is in your breath, and by breathing with more awareness, you reach into your deeper self and become more in touch with yourself. Awareness of your breath connects you with the power of your soul, and allows your mind and body to respond with more clarity, focus, and groundedness.

The poses that connect to the *Heih* are the Extended Hand-to-Knee Pose and the Extended Hand-to-Big-Toe Pose. When coming into these *Heih* poses, we need stability, balance, and flow in our breath. The inhale is at the lifting of the leg with the hand on the knee, or holding the big toe or foot, as you keep steady and lift with your spine. The exhale is the grounding on the supporting leg. It is your connection to the Earth, the soil that breathes this infinite life, drawing deep breath from your heart into the supporting and extended leg, the foundation of your body.

The lifted leg symbolizes the balance of energy in your inhalations, while the supporting leg stands firmly on the ground and draws steadiness in your exhalations. The sages tell us that the openness of the *Heih* resembles an entrance where the energy of breath passes through from within and surrounding the body. The *Heih* poses also remind us of our freedom and power to choose a path we wish for when we stand strong and free.

The letter *Heih* is formed by three lines. It has a vertical and a horizontal line attached at one corner, and a third short line on the other side. Kabalah explains that the horizontal line represents the mind, and the vertical line represents the expression of the heart. The short line is the action we do to inspire positive intentions. The shape of the *Heih* teaches us that if there is harmony in the heart and mind, then there is freedom in the body and soul. The space between the short line (action) and the horizontal line (mind) remind us to see the energy between each breath and to pause to make space for the action to be inspiring. For this reason, the opening below the *Heih* is the creative space from which we can experience free expression. As in the *Heih*, the Earth's creative energy is such that it causes seeds planted in the ground to grow. When we cultivate our breath, we grow deeply from the soil of our body and into our soul.

Body

Poses:

Extended Hand-to-Knee Pose

Extended Hand-to-Big-Toe Pose

Extended Hand-to-Knee Pose

Create the kavana (*intention*):

Envision your breath as the universe breathing into your root and blossoming into your body.

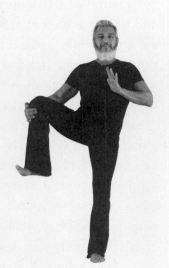

Directions into the pose:

1. Stand in Mountain Pose.

2. Breathe in; breathe out. Feel the extension of your whole body.

3. Gaze into a point in front of you and shift all your weight to your left leg.

4. As you press the four corners of your foot (the mounds of your large and small toes and the sides of your heel) into the ground, inhale, and lift your right knee to the level of your hip.

5. Exhale, and feel your standing leg strong and rooted.

6. Stay here or continue on to Extended Hand-to-Knee Pose.

7. Open your hip by bringing your knee to the right. Place your left hand on your left hip to keep your stability.

8. Feel strong and balanced by engaging your core and focusing on the movement and rhythm of your breath. You are bringing harmony into your body.

9. Hold for a few breaths.

10. Place your left hand at your heart, in half prayer position.

11. Press your shoulders down and away from your ears.

12. Hold for a few breaths, working to feel tremendous stability and groundedness.

13. Lower your foot to the floor. Repeat on the other side.

Health and benefits:

- Opens the hips
- Stretches the muscles between the shoulder blades and the neck
- Strengthens the backs of the legs while also toning the core
- Improves balance

Extended Hand-to-Big-Toe Pose

Create the kavana (*intention*):

Envision yourself breathing from the air of the Earth, rising into your supporting leg and into your body.

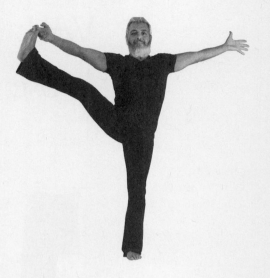

Directions into the pose:

1. From the Extended Hand-to-Knee Pose, reconnect to your breath as you soften your gaze.

2. Bring your right knee back to the center and grab your big toe.

3. Inhale, and begin to extend your leg forward while maintaining a long upper body.

4. Open your leg to the right and extend the opposite arm out to the left.

5. Gaze at your fingers, and think of the energy of *hayin* and *hayin de'hayin* passing through you and crossing over. Bring your leg back and lower your foot to the floor.

6. Repeat on the other side.

Health and benefits:

- Same as above

CHAPTER 6

VAV: Alignment

Pose: Mountain

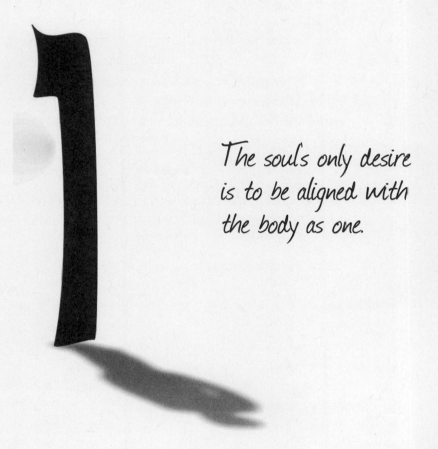

The soul's only desire is to be aligned with the body as one.

The *Vav* corresponds to the English letters V and W and has a numerical value of 6.

Soul

Vav: V'Ani Eheyeh L'Olam. "I am forever eternal."

—Akivah

A story is told about a prince who had a crooked spine. Each time he went out in public, he felt insecure due to his bent posture. One day, the prince had the idea to meet with the best sculptor, and he assigned the sculptor to make an image of him, but with a straight back. Finally, after months passed, the statue was finished. It was declared by the entire palace as a masterpiece. Everyone suggested placing it somewhere public for all to see. The prince, however, chose to display it in a secret garden near the palace where only he could appreciate its beauty. Once installed, the prince would often escape to this mini-paradise and spend hours gazing, meditating, and shaping into this image of himself. A strange thing happened: people began to notice that the prince was not as crooked as before. Rumors spread that the prince was appearing more handsome and royal. When this news got to the prince, he rejoiced and continued to go to his secret garden more fervently to shape into the image of himself until his spine had become perfectly straight, and he had transformed into the prince of his dreams.

How many of us dream to heal from our difficulties? To become our best version possible?

The Letter

The sages describe the letter *Vav* as an image of an upright man made up of many layers, both physical and spiritual, all of which exist individually and perfectly. If we have awareness and determination, we can bring all our qualities together to form an aligned body and soul. The vertical *Vav* reminds us to search inward like the prince and discover our true potential, trusting that, with effort, we can reshape ourselves into a divine image. Unlike animals, Adam was made upright because he was created in "the divine image," says the book of Genesis (chapter 1).

We all have an image in our mind of the Creator. I remember as a young boy having a discussion with my friends about the Creator, describing him as a mighty and powerful old wise man with a long white beard, sitting high on a throne governing the world. As adults, our understanding of the Creator becomes more complex and varied because our feelings and perceptions of the Creator are affected by the attitudes and opinions of family, friends, courses we take, books we read, and all heard and shared experiences.

How are we in the image the Creator? Is the Creator a she or a he? In reality, the Creator is taking on the role of both a father who provides life and a mother who conceives seeds of life and embraces them with love. The book of Genesis states that the first man was created as one human having both male and female features. This being was then divided in two, as it is written in Genesis (chapter 1), "The Creator made man in His image...both male and female, He created them." The initial human consisted of physical features and qualities that would shape the eventual characteristics of both men and women.

Humankind is the reflection of the Creator both physically and spiritually. If the universe is indeed holographic, as many physicists speculate, then we are a hologram of some projection by the Creator. In essence, he is everything, and everything is her.

Everything that exists in the soul is the Creator dwelling within us. He exists inside the body, activating each thought, word, and action. The body and the soul, together, carry the qualities that make us both physical and spiritual. We are spiritual beings having physical experiences. No person on this planet can ever be just one or the other because being both is essential to experiencing life. If either the soul or the body were missing, we would cease to exist.

At our essence—past our appearance, skin, flesh, muscles, and bones—is a common alignment deriving from the same root. Horizontally, our soul expressions may vary in the way our body flows. It is only in our physical expression of this essence that we are different from one another. Vertically, however, our souls flow from, and resemble, the same root of all souls.

Our families, cultures, nations, and circumstances develop us into the unique people we become. Our personal history affects who we eventually become as individuals. Some of us will become deeply attached to our culture and origins, while others will be more remote, perhaps detached, and often secularized. A few will find peace in their heart by embracing a spirituality different from what they were exposed to in childhood. Those who practice religion will have had the taste of honoring the sacred days and rituals of their ancestors. Others outside religion will honor life as the supreme consciousness or as the natural order of things. They will cultivate their essence in a unique way that brings awareness to the energetic enfolding and unfolding of life. Depending on how significant your circumstances are and the contracts you signed up for in this life's purpose, your image of the Creator will influence who you are and how you think, act, and speak.

Thought is our inner garment and the seed from which intention is emanated from the soul. Speech and action, our ways of expressing intention, are the garments. Positive intention comes from the soil of supreme consciousness, from where the light of nothing, and of everything, shines brilliantly.

The soul is revealed when good intention fills us with inspiration and lifts our lives to the highest spiritual level. Here, you open yourself to the greatest possibilities, while remaining strongly rooted in your actual situation. Your intention will determine the quality of your actions. How much of your soul will be put into your deeds? Will you reach out to someone in need out of duty or because you sincerely care and want to make a positive difference in that person's life?

Sublime intention is reached when your intent is aligned with the universal intent to bring light into the world, when you find harmony in body and soul, and when you improve the world by your actions.

The letter *Vav* offers us a way of aligning our center of energy with the divine image. The *Vav* represents the *sefirot*, the spiritual channels within the body that balance the flow of energy that moves between our thoughts, emotions, and bodies.

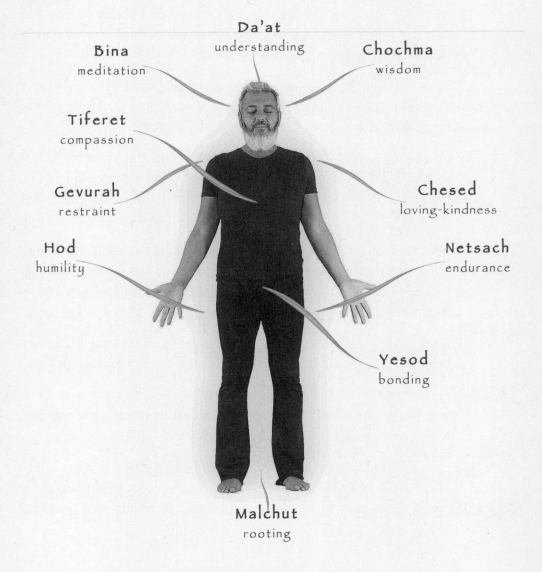

Da'at
understanding

Bina
meditation

Chochma
wisdom

Tiferet
compassion

Gevurah
restraint

Chesed
loving-kindness

Hod
humility

Netsach
endurance

Yesod
bonding

Malchut
rooting

Each of the *sefirot* shines with a unique glow of its own. The *sefirot* also overlap each other to create a multitude of character and personality. What you perceive will affect how you view your life. Perception is projection and will determine your level of clarity and how you see the Creator. Ultimately, what you believe will motivate you to tap into your soul and awaken your inner powers that can shape the world around you as you desire.

The *sefirot* are like the *chakras* in Eastern medicine ("wheels" of energy in the body), aligned in a vertical line of seven levels of maturation that can be experienced.

1. Loving-kindness (*chesed*), located on the right side of the upper body, is the most important foundation of our relationships because it involves both giving and receiving.

2. Restraint (*gevurah*), on the left side, is our focus and ability to love and share it according to what is needed. Restraint gives us the awareness needed when we shine our light upon others.

3. Compassion (*tiferet*), in the center of the heart, allows us to have a deeper understanding of love and how to show it warmly and deeply to others. Compassion is the balance between love and restraint.

4. Endurance (*netsach*) is located on the right side of the lower body. It is the belief that deep inside, there is a spiritual warrior yearning to shine and inspire us to go further. It is the strength of the mind and body that we can cultivate when there is a fiery heart leading the way.

5. Humility (*hod*), on the left side of the lower body, is the inner silence and gratitude that makes us conscious of our divine abilities. It offers modesty that comes from the realization that there is so much to learn and so much growth to achieve.

6. Bonding (*yesod*), at the level of the sexual organs and underneath, is connecting deeply with our sense of creativity and sharing our energies with another.

7. Rooting (*malchut*) is the foundational platform at the level of the feet, from which our energies will arise and grow.

As with the chakras, within each *sefira* (the singular form of *sefirot*) exists a spiritual challenge that must be overcome. Within each energy field exists information that will help us grow spiritually and physically. By refining the quality of the information found at each level, we improve our personality and reactions. The more we gain from each of these energies, the further will we elevate our intellectual and emotional powers and our physical body, and the better will we channel our responses to life.

The mind also has an alignment referred to by the Alter Rebbe as the three brains.[6] They are comprised of *chochma*, "wisdom and ideas," on the right side of the brain; *bina*, or "meditation," on the left side; and *da'at*, or "understanding," at the third eye at the center of the forehead. *Da'at* allows us to internalize ideas of the mind and feelings of the heart, and influences our perceptions and reactions to our environments. The *Vav* brings harmony within as we connect with others and share our inner being. Because we come from a higher light, it is in our nature to desire to come closer to each other and connect to more light.

Each decision or choice we make will elicit a certain energy that will be imprinted into the memory of our body and mind. When we begin to view ourselves through the alignment of the *Vav*, we develop lenses for each of the *sefirot* and the three brains, and we start to view and reach for the hidden powers within us and transcend our limitations. We expand our mind, open our heart, and stretch our body to levels that are reached only when the unconscious is released. By directing our personal channels of energy, we can benefit positively from all information that enters and exits our mind, body, breath, and soul.

To live meaningfully requires an awakening of our energy channels. The soul needs to be cared for just as the body does. The soul also functions vertically, as does our physique. Understanding your body will allow you to achieve harmony between your physical and spiritual self. Connecting to your soul leads you to discovering the power behind each breath you take as you open yourself to greater life in thoughts, feelings, and actions.

If you want your yoga practice to be internalized more deeply, you must reach beyond the tissue and bones of your body and touch your essence by caring for your soul—the piece of the Creator inside of you.

The shape of each Hebrew letter opens to these channels of energy found within the *Vav*, and brings rejuvenation. When you see your body as a vessel for light, your mind as a tool for meditation, and your heart as an altar for feeling and embracing, you will have grasped the very power that constantly creates and energizes you to bring greater happiness, love, focus, beauty, strength, humility, depth, stability, and unity into your life.

Breath: Energetic Shape and Intention

The kavanas *of the Vav are feelings of gratefulness, stability, alignment of body, and openness to your channels of energy. It is awareness of the Earth, sky, and life that embraces you.*

The *Vav* requires rootedness in your body, openness in your mind, and flow in your breath. The inhale is the connection you make to the Earth as you press down through the four corners of your feet. It is at the extension of the arms overhead or at the placing of hands to the heart, the lengthening from the inside, and the expansion of the heart energy as it rises to the crown of your head and joins the energy above you. Exhale while maintaining the uplifting energy of the inhale, and melt down through the body, releasing all tensions and deepening to your core's center. The exhale is in the feet, where you are rooted and create space for your energy channels to be activated.

The sages teach that the vertical shape of the *Vav* symbolizes our own upright posture. While the lower part of the letter represents the feet firmly planted on Earth, the upper part is the alignment of the torso as the head reaches softly toward heaven. The shape of the *Vav*—also called *Tadasana* in Sanskrit, or the Mountain Pose—reflects your ability to be rooted on Earth and yet connected to the energy above you, heaven.

In Mountain Pose, we lengthen our body from the ground to the sky and seek to increase space within our being through breath. Every exhale draws us deeper into the Earth, while our inhales bring us closer to the sky. In *Tadasana* (which aims for a perfect alignment of the spine, feet, arms, shoulders, and head), our whole being stretches along a line of energy, which reminds us to be present in the moment. This standing pose prepares the body for groundedness and awareness in the practice of the other postures.

The *Vav* is similar to the word "and." Its function as a letter is to unite words and ideas to form sentences, paragraphs, and chapters. Similarly, *Tadasana* joins postures together in a flow in the beginning, anywhere in a practice, or at the end. In yoga, we often begin our practice by standing in *Tadasana*. *Tadasana* is also a transition pose between *asanas* (Sanskrit for "posture") as we flow into sequences in our yoga practice. *Tadasana* is not only about feeling grounded; it also is an *asana* that connects the entire practice into a unified whole.

In Sanskrit, *tada* means "mountain." In Hebrew, *tada*, pronounced as "todah," means "thank you." I often refer to *Tadasana* as the Thank You Pose. When standing in this pose, bring your palms together in a prayer and think *Todah!* (*Thank you!*) Be thankful for the life you have and the opportunities you have been given. Think of the hands together as a symbol of gratefulness for being alive and having this moment to join your soul together in perfect harmony with the Creator's soul. The ten fingers and toes remind us of the seven *sefirot*, energy channels, along with the three brains that can be tapped into while doing the *Vav* pose.

When standing in the *Vav* position, envision becoming a channel of energy that flows through your intentions into feelings and actions.

In the Hero Pose, which takes the body of *Vav*, the intention is to draw your channels of light into *malchut*, "the energy underneath you," and cause all your qualities to grow.

Body

Poses:

Mountain Pose

Hero's Pose Grabbing for Opposite Elbows

Hero's Pose with Arms Outstretched

Mountain Pose

Create the kavana *(intention):*

You are a vertical channel connecting to your energy channels rising. This pose helps improve your posture, balance, and focus.

Directions into the pose:

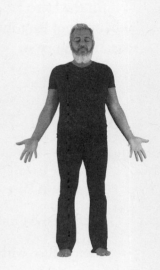

1. Stand with your feet parallel and draw an imaginary line extending from between your feet to the top of your head.

2. Root the four corners of your feet firmly into the ground, lift your thighs up, and spiral the tops of them inward.

3. Focus forward and center your body and mind into a common flow of breath.

4. Retain an open chest and lifted heart.

5. Connect to the energy rising in the inner legs toward the pelvis.

6. Tuck your tailbone, draw the belly up and in, and lengthen your spine upward.

7. Feel the crown of your head reaching away from the spine as it ascends toward heaven.

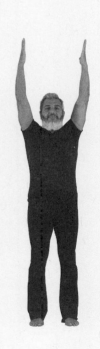

8. You can stay here and enjoy. To go further, inhale, and extend your arms into the sky with your palms facing each other, energetically reaching upward.

9. Grow taller from your earthly roots and connect to your spiritual ones.

10. On an exhale, lower your arms to your sides.

11. Position your shoulders above the hips, roll them back, and place your arms by your sides, palms facing the sides of the body.

Health and benefits:

- Benefits posture and aligns the spine
- Opens the chest and heart
- Works the core by toning the abdominals and buttocks
- Relaxes the body, enhances focus, and creates determination

Hero's Pose Grabbing for Opposite Elbows

Create the kavana *(intention):*

You are a vessel connecting to the energy of the Earth. This pose stretches the thighs and ankles, and improves posture.

Directions into the pose:

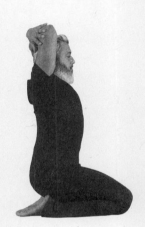

1. Kneel on the ground with your knees and inner legs together and your feet about twenty inches apart.

2. Rest your buttocks on the ground between your feet, with your toes pointing backward.

3. Press the tops of your feet into the ground.

4. Connect your body to the energy underneath you as it rises into the back of your heart.

5. Lift your arms to the sky, and envision connecting your channels of energy into the soil of awareness. Grab the opposite elbows above your head.

6. Remain in this position for a few breaths.

Health and benefits:

- Great for meditation and pranayama
- Stretches the thighs, quadriceps, hamstrings, and ankles
- Relieves pain or discomfort in the lower back

Hero's Pose with Arms Outstretched

Create the kavana *(intention):*

You are a channel connecting the energy of the Earth to beyond. This pose helps open the knees and lengthens the spine.

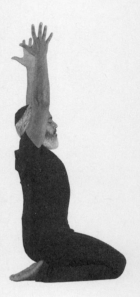

Directions into the pose:

1. Repeat the steps of the Hero's Pose above up to the point of grabbing for opposite elbows.

2. Inhale, and stretch your arms above your head, fingers pointing away from you.

3. Exhale, and feel the beautiful flow of life moving from your fingertips into the Earth.

4. Hold as long as you can, continuing to breathe deeply and evenly.

Health and benefits:

*   Same as above

CHAPTER 7

ZAYIN: Shabbat

Pose: Side Plank

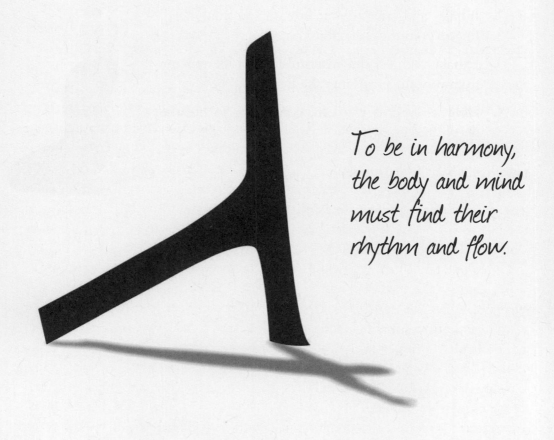

To be in harmony, the body and mind must find their rhythm and flow.

The *Zayin* corresponds to the English letters X and Z and has a numerical value of 7.

Soul

Zayin: Zan Ume-Farness Kol Yetsurei Kapav. "He sustains all shapes made from his hands."

—Akivah

Friday evening in our home is the climax of the week. For twenty-five hours, from Friday night at sunset until Saturday at nightfall, I do not write, drive a car, flick on the lights, use my computer, use my cell phone, or engage in everyday activities that involve using fire or electricity. I also abstain from any form of work or labor that could involve my body or mind. Instead, I spend the day resting and detaching from my daily chores in order to focus on nourishing my soul spiritually.

This weekly ritual that I honor is a tradition that dates back to Creation. According to the Bible, thousands of years ago, when the Creator began making the world on the first Sunday, he finished shaping everything in heaven and on Earth by the sixth day—Friday. And on the seventh day, Saturday, the numerical value of *Zayin*, he paused to meditate in stillness on all that he had done. The *Zayin* rest tells us that our abstinence from performing our regular activities is essential for our movement forward. *Shabbat* is a time in our busy schedules to unplug, disconnect from a hectic life, and take a moment to nurture that inner flame.

This practice of observing *shabbat* is embraced by countless people worldwide, as too is the custom of lighting candles on Friday night at sunset, in honor of *shabbat*. Lighting candles for the *shabbat* is a reminder that the soul is like a flame, constantly rising high and connecting to its source. Everything that exists in the soul (the inner flame) also exists within the body (the carrier of the flame). The body and soul together hold the qualities that make us alive. To be alive means we are constantly pulsing our breath in and out, and expanding and contracting from within.

A flame is produced by combining oil with a wick. Both the oil and the wick are combustible, even though separately they could never produce light. For the soul's light to be revealed, a combination of elements is needed: a mind to meditate on its wisdom, a heart to feel its warmth, a mouth to speak about its truth, and hands and feet to experience and share its beauty.

There is a particular Kabalistic body flow that we perform when lighting the candles of *shabbat*. As the candles are lit, we gaze at the flames for a moment, then move our arms around the flames several times as if we are drawing their light into our body. Some people flow five times to arouse the five levels of our soul, known in Hebrew as *kochos*, meaning powers of the soul, similar to the *koshas* in yoga—the five "sheaths," or layers, of the body. These levels are the forces that we tap into in order to gain a sense of wholeness in our lives.[7] The levels, in order from the outermost to the innermost, are as follows:

1. *Nefesh*, the part of the soul most connected to the body, related to your physical responses to life

2. *Ruach*, the spirit that manifests itself through your emotional reactions

3. *Neshamah*, the wisdom to distinguish right from wrong, enabling you to discover a path in life that is meaningful

4. *Chaya*, the life-force found in your energy centers, known in Hebrew as *sefirot*, meaning "channels of light"

5. *Yechidah*, the highest level that can be reached for the true self to experience bliss and harmony. At the level of *yechida*, like the *shabbat* flame, balance is reached when your *kochos*, "powers of the soul," are aligned into one active force that brings illumination into all of your life.

The Letter

The *Zayin* teaches us that *shabbat* is the flame that brings illumination to every moment of our lives. When *shabbat* arrives, all things around us pause so we may examine their inner workings. Is the inside of the flame burning? Is it warm? Bright? A flame moves with thirst to reach upward, as if to detach itself from the wick and connect to something much greater, purer, and more spiritual. Still, it pulls back to its body, to the Earth, assuming its function to be a source of illumination within the physical realm.

We all yearn to find those rare instances of stillness—times when we can replenish our energy by opening to the light within and letting go to receive. At the core of the *Zayin* is simply being yourself, without attachment whatsoever to anything or anyone. *Zayin* is the secret of stillness the Creator called the *shabbat*—the moment of just being still—and made on the seventh day of Creation.

Finding sacredness in the moment is dependent upon what we do with our time. We often sacrifice time to gain material possessions. Sacredness does not come from the accumulation of material things, but from the creation of inspirational instances that eternally uplift us, beyond space or time. How do we make time sacred? There is a reality in time where the purpose is not to have but to just be, not to control, but to share, not to conquer, but to surrender. The Torah says, "Six days a week, create in space. On the *Zayin* (seventh day), the *shabbat*, step back, look inward, meditate, and create sacredness within time."[8] We therefore come to stillness when we slow down the breath, look inward, release any attachment whatsoever, and let go of space to be present.

Resting Pose, called *Shavasana* in Sanskrit, is like *shabbat* in that it is about letting go. In Hebrew, *Shavasana* consists of two words: *shavas*, meaning "rest," and *ana*, meaning "I am." *Shavas* is spelled with the letters—*Shin, Beit* (pronounced as *Veit*), and *Tav* (pronounced as *Sav*)—that spell *shabbat*. I mentioned in the introduction that each of these Hebrew letters has a softer sound variation. The *Shin* (SH) is also *Sien* (SS), the *Beit* (B) is *Veit* (V), and the *Tav* is *Sav* (S). The soft variations of these letters speak of the unique state of tranquility we can achieve when coming into the stillness of *shabbat*.

What is rest? *Shabbat* is creating a moment to be deeply attached to your inner world by detaching from the outer world. *Shabbat* is a way of drawing deeper into yoga, and will be found at every level of your practice. When you begin your yoga practice, start to relax and meditate, center yourself by taking a deep breath, and pause before exhaling. You will achieve calmness by being yourself and knowing who you really are. The stillness is allowing your essence to take over. Experience the moment of awareness. Be here and now. When you let go of your thoughts and limitations, you can envision the space you created inside. Look inward. As you inhale, imagine that you are drawing from the breath of life, and as you exhale, imagine that you are sharing your breath with all of life. Stay in this space for a moment.

As you begin to flow in your practice, envision yourself going deeper into your body and drawing into this inner life. When you come into the poses, continue to meditate on your movements. Become aware of the pulsation of your breath, in and out, and as you draw downward, lift up, contract, and expand. Search for the stillness within the flow. As you flow into your practice, connect to your heart. Find your presence.

Breath: Energetic Shape and Intention

The kavanas of the Zayin are feelings of lightness, gracefulness, stability, alignment of body and Earth, relaxation, and openness to your channels of energy. It is awareness of the energy surrounding you, below you, and above you.

The *Zayin* requires balance, openness in your mind, and steadiness in your breath moving like a wave in the ocean. The Side Plank Poses concentrate on one arm drawing light from above, while the other arm transmits the light to the Earth. The idea of one supporting leg planted to the Earth and the other extended to the back is to show that while we connect to the Earth, we also root into the energy surrounding us.

In the Half Moon Pose, the inhale is the lifting action and comes from your center, extending energy from within to the whole body. It is also the extension out from the heart. The horizontal lengthening from the inside goes from the extended-leg toes to the crown of the head and the expansion of the heart as it shines out to the sides. The posture reminds us that balance in our body comes when there is harmony between the energy underneath us and the energy surrounding us. The exhale is on the settling down of the supporting leg and the fingers to the Earth, rooting down through the corners of your supporting foot reaching toward your center, wrapped by the core.

The *Zayin* pose is also assumed by lying down, as in Resting Pose (lying on your back with palms facing upward). The direction of the pose is to melt down into the Earth and receive the energy cultivated during the practice.

But *shabbat* is not just about resting, and neither is the Resting Pose. It is harmony between your body and soul as you bond with the energy underneath and above you. You become the heartbeat of the ground as your soul opens itself to the sky.

Body

Poses:

Side Plank Pose

Side Plank Pose with Elbow on Ground

Side Plank Pose with One Foot on Ground

Half Moon Pose

Resting Pose (Shavasana)

Side Plank Pose

Create the kavana (*intention*):

Envision yourself as a ray of light carrying energy between Earth and heaven.

Directions into the pose:

1. Begin in Downward Dog. Exhale and come into a high push-up position.

2. Spin your heels to the left and reach your right hand up toward the sky, making sure your left hand is directly beneath your left shoulder.

3. Stack your feet together and place your upper hip over your lower hip.

4. Engage actively through all muscles of your body. From the crown of your head to the tips of your toes, you should feel one long line of free-flowing energy.

5. Visualize two lines of traction being created: from the crown of your head to the soles of your feet and from the palm pressing into the ground to your fingertips reaching to the sky.

6. Alternatively, bring your lower knee down to the Earth.

7. To close, come back to high push-up and repeat on the other side.

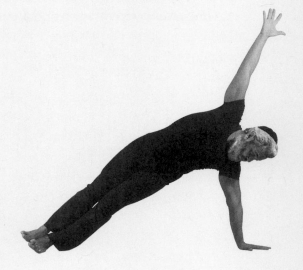

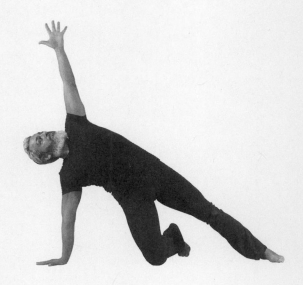

Health and benefits:

- Stretches the arms and the wrists
- Stretches and strengthens the front and back of the torso
- Tones the legs, arms, and abdomen
- Improves sense of balance
- Improves concentration and focus

Side Plank Pose with Elbow on Ground

Create the kavana (*intention*):

Visualize your body being raised from the Earth as you connect to the sky.

Directions into the pose:

1. Follow the same instructions in the Side Plank above except at step #2, place your elbow instead of your hand on the Earth.

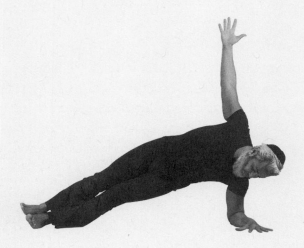

Health and benefits:

• Same as above

Side Plank Pose with One Foot on Ground

Createthe kavana (intention):

Visualize your body lifting the energy from underneath you to the sky above you.

Directions into the pose:

1. Follow the same instructions for Side Plank Pose except at step #2, place one foot on the Earth in front of your other leg instead of stacking it on the other foot.

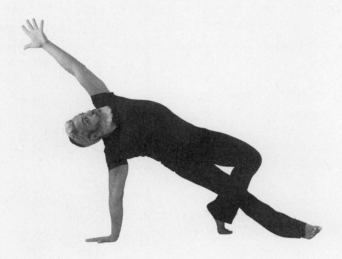

Health and benefits:

- Same as above

Half Moon Pose

Create the kavana (*intention*):

Visualize that while your supporting leg roots down, your extended leg roots into the surrounding energy.

Directions into the pose:

1. Step your feet wide apart.

2. Inhale, and extend your arms out to the sides.

3. Turn your front foot forward so it's parallel to the long edge of your mat, and turn your back foot in. (You can also begin from Triangle Pose where your upper body is moving forward, while one hand rests on the front hip.)

4. Exhale, bend your front knee, and slide your back foot forward along the Earth.

5. Inhale, and extend your front hand forward, under your shoulder.

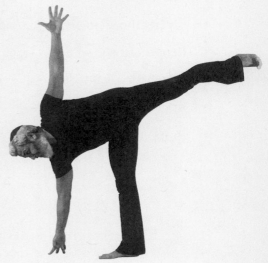

6. Exhale, and press your front fingertips and standing heel firmly into the ground, while straightening this supporting leg. Simultaneously lift the back leg toward the sky.

7. Move your body weight mostly onto the supporting leg while pressing your hand softly to the Earth as you establish balance.

8. Open your chest, and lengthen your neck and spine.

9. Envision drawing energy from the Earth into the supporting leg through the standing groin.

10. Extend through the heel and maintain strength in the lifted leg.

11. Press the sacrum firmly toward the back torso, and lengthen the coccyx toward the lifted heel.

12. Connect to the energy surrounding your body.

13. Gaze at one spot, and breathe with awareness to a firmly rooted standing leg as well as a firm and extended outstretched leg.

14. Keep the knee of your supporting leg unlocked and your kneecap aligned forward.

15. Rotate your upper body to the side, upper hip steadily reaching forward.

16. Repeat on the other side.

Health and benefits:

- Improves balance and coordination
- Creates focus and relieves stress
- Stretches the hamstrings, calves, and groin
- Strengthens the arches, ankles, knees, and thighs
- Opens the shoulders, chest, and hips
- Lengthens the spine
- Strengthens the core and buttocks
- Roots the ankles and thighs
- Builds focus and willpower

Resting Pose (Shavasana)

Create the kavana (*intention*):

Envision a line of energy from the crown of your head extending to the soles of your feet. In *Shavasana*, the body is released completely to the Earth, while the mind is clear and the heart is open, allowing the practice to be internalized.

Directions into the pose:

1. Get what you need to be comfortable to lie on your back and relax your body.

2. Allow your legs to part slightly and your toes to roll to the sides.

3. Rest your arms to the sides, equidistant from the body.

4. Place your shoulder blades flat on the ground and underneath you, and tuck your tailbone.

5. Breath slowly and softly. Let each breath melt your body into the Earth.

6. Open yourself to *shavas* and *ana*, "I am rest," and feel completely and peacefully at one.

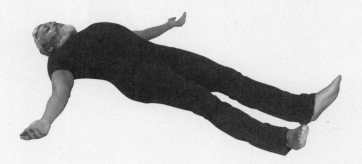

Health and benefits:

- Teaches you to relax and to breathe

- Relieves symptoms related to fatigue, including jet lag

- Restores blood pressure and the respiratory system to a healthy balance

- Lowers blood pressure

- Calms the brain and releases stress

CHAPTER 8

CHEIT: Energy
Pose: The Wheel

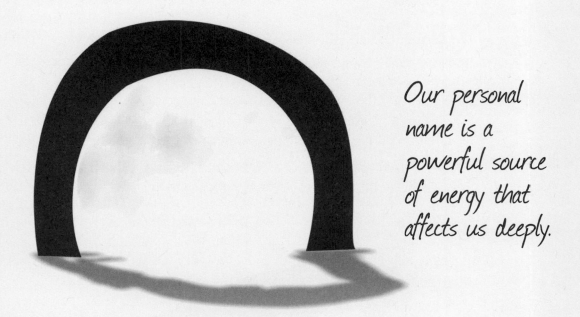

Our personal name is a powerful source of energy that affects us deeply.

The *Cheit* corresponds to the English letters *CH* and has a numerical value of 8.

Soul

Cheit: Sheburei Lev Chavivin. "An open heart is a desirous space."

—Akivah

I come from a line of boys named Yehuda. This is the sacred name my father gave me after his father, who was so named by his father after his grandfather, and so on. Although I am better known by most people as Audi, my sacred name, Yehuda, is used by my spiritual teachers and colleagues of Kabalah, and when I am called to read from the Torah during ceremonial prayers.

What makes a name special is its meaning and the meanings of the Hebrew letters that form it. Similar to the way the world was created through the sacred shapes and powerful words, each letter of your name brings out a certain energy in your soul that affects your body and character.

The sages say that the inspiration we get in naming our children is prophetic, as it comes from the supreme consciousness and reaches deeply into our essence. Certainly, as parents, we may have been inspired by something we read, a family member who passed on, or someone we look up to. Whatever the reason is, when we choose a specific name, it draws from a higher level of creativity that comes to us at special moments when an important decision must be made. This choice influences the name the parent will give to the soul that has just entered the body of the child and powerfully influences the child throughout their life.

If we look closely at the word "soul" in Hebrew, *neshamah,* we notice that the word "name" in Hebrew, *shem,* is spelled with the two middle letters of the word—*Shin* and *Mem*—telling us that the energy of one's name comes from the center of that person's soul. Your soul enters your body from the breath of the Creator breathing into your nostrils. The name you have been given represents a code specific for unlocking the connection of your body and soul. Because your name is so powerful, it will influence the way you live your life and see the world inside and outside of you. During your physical lifetime, your name will come to symbolize who you are, what you do, and how you are perceived. The sages explain that when we finish our mission on Earth and ascend on high to be face-to-face with our maker, we will be asked if we lived according to our name.

My sacred name has an old history. According to tradition, the first-ever recorded Yehuda was the fourth son of Jacob, the biblical patriarch. When he was born, the reaction his mother Leah had was, "Now I will praise the Creator," with the Hebrew word for praise—*audeh*—which is the root of the word *Yehuda.*[9] His mother named him Yehuda to bring out the qualities of praise, honor, and gratitude as personal attributes to be achieved.

His father, Jacob, envisioned that royalty would come from his son, and so he blessed Yehuda to possess the strength of a *gur aryeh*, a young courageous lion. From Yehuda came the tribe of Judah, known to be the most powerful among his brothers, who together became the twelve tribes of Israel. Yehuda is depicted by the image of a lion—*aryeh*—and from whom the monarchies of Israel descended, such as King David and his son, King Solomon, both representing the lion of Judah.

The sages explain that after Adam had named every animal and creature on Earth, he meditated on their nature and shapes, and saw the forms of the letters that guided him in their naming. He named the animals first in *Leshon Hakodesh,* the sacred language of the Creator (afterward interpreting each name into seventy other languages). When Adam named the lion *aryeh*, he combined the letters *Alef, Yud,* and *Heih* from the Creator's name, envisioning that the lion would be the king of all animals. He added the letter *Reish* for *ruach,* "the divine breath," within him, so that when the lion would roar (as in the sound of *Reish*), all would know that they were in the presence of royalty. He named the horse *sus* because of its joy and exultation in its movement, which is the meaning of the word *sus* in Hebrew. The donkey was named *chamor* because of his heaviness and slowness to move, which is the meaning of *chamor.* Adam named each animal and species by meditating and reflecting on its character, movement, and power.

When Adam had finished naming the animals, he then named the woman that the Creator had made Eve. In Hebrew, it is pronounced as "chaya," a short form of *Chayout,* deriving from the letter *Cheit,* meaning "the source of life." Eve was named as such because she was destined to be the root mother of humankind by bearing the children who would start the world. The Creator then turned to Adam and said, "Now name me!"

Adam reflected on how the Creator was truly the essence of creation both physically and spiritually. He named the Creator *Adonai,* "the Master." Adonai is really not so much a name as it is a character, referring to one who is mighty and great. A powerful leader or seer may also be called Adonai if he or she has the skills of a visionary that sees the whole and its details deeply, without ever losing sight of one or the other. Adonai is a king, queen, provider, teacher, father, mother, and friend to the people he or she oversees.

When it was time, however, to name himself, man was at a loss. After pondering, he named himself Adam, symbolizing that he came from the Earth—*adamah*—and that he was created in the image of the Creator—*adameh.*

The Letter

The *Cheit* teaches us about awareness by connecting to our inner self through the meaning of our personal name. When we develop our perception, we become more sensitive to the flow of energy and the uniqueness of each form of life. The power of the *Cheit* lies in the idea that each person or thing is spiritually interconnected through a circular energy, the shape of the letter that moves to and from ourselves and toward others, creating a bond of light.

The letters that spell your name have special meaning. You can connect to the code of your soul by meditating on the meaning of your name and by shaping your body into the letters of your name.

The letter *Yud* of my name, Yehuda, reminds me to always remain humble no matter how great my achievements may be; the *Heih*, that I should cultivate awareness of my breath; the *Vav*, to live life fully as I ground myself in all areas; the *Dalet*, that I should be conscious of my words and seek to speak positively no matter what.

Hearing your name over and over again each time someone calls you has the effect of awakening inner feelings triggered by the sounds made from the letters of your name that have special meaning.

I remember the first time I did the yoga postures of my name Audi; the feeling was powerful. As I moved from Warrior II to Warrior III and Forward Bend, my heart opened to feelings of gratitude and freedom, and was open to receiving and sharing. From the oneness of the *Alef* in the Warrior II Pose, I meditated upon how it was essential to be both grounded and physical, and yet be above ground and more spiritual. The steadiness of the *Vav*, as in the Mountain Pose, made me feel more focused and strong. The reaching out in *Dalet*, performed in the Warrior III Pose, told me that I can be balanced when I reach out and be there for others. The all-embracing feeling of the *Yud*, as in the Forward Bend, allowed me to internalize these energies alluded to in my name.

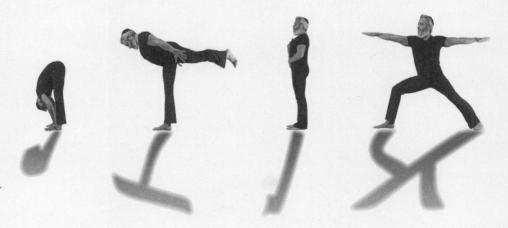

Names are hidden codes that have different meanings depending upon how the Hebrew letters are combined. Your name becomes the channel that reflects the essence of who you are and the character that you possess. Because the letters are the sacred shapes that brought creation, they carry hidden energies that you can tap into to discover the essence of your name.

Discovering the letters through yoga, your body will tap into a spiritual creativity that reaches into you deeply. Give it a try! When you start to discover the Hebrew letters in meaning, breath, and postures, you will learn the sacred shapes through the ABCs I have matched with each Hebrew letter. You can then develop a flow where you move your body into the shapes that spell your name, and feel deeply connected to yourself as you practice. The flow of your name can be part of your self-practice or done when you feel the need to draw inward into your essence and soul.

Breath: Energetic Shape and Intention

The kavanas of the Cheit are feelings of the life-force passing through you, energy in the body, sacredness in your name, openness in your heart to feel deeply, harmony in body and soul, and light and fire in the heart.

The *Cheit* requires focus, harmony, suppleness in spine, being grounded, and strength. The inhale, as in the Wheel Pose, is at the pressing of palms on the Earth as the torso is lifted. The inhale is also at the pressing down of the feet as the body rises into an arch. The exhale is at the settling of the body as you rise higher. It is also the shining through the heart as your elbows draw back and your chest draws forward. The exhale is the gathering of the energy underneath you as you draw light from the Earth through the hands and feet into the heart.

An interesting image you can cultivate when coming into the Wheel Pose is a teaching from Ezekiel the prophet, who envisions animals and humans as "moving as wheels within wheels," their bodies, breath, and spirit flowing with grace in circles, turning the wheels of light higher and higher.[10]

The Reverse Table Top Pose has its inhale at the lifting of the hips as you press into the hands and feet. The exhale is at the rooting down, as you maintain a lengthened tailbone extended from the core.

When shaping your body into the *Cheit*, your feet and hands become the symbol of the Earth, and the more rooted you are, the more your body will rise and your heart will shine out.

Your heart is the window for connecting to your life-force, as your body and soul root into the one light. With your heart, you can navigate deep feelings and intentions, and go deeper into yourself through cultivating *kavana* based on learning the meanings of the letters that spell your name. The letter *Cheit* means "vitality," and in each person and in all things, it can be found within its name.

The Hassidic masters explain that there are two levels to the *Cheit* life-force: the "essential life" and the "potential life."[11] The essential energy is what allows us to exist and function daily through our body, mind, and heart. The potential energy is a reservoir of energy normally dormant, but that comes out when we awaken it by cultivating the life-force within us. Each person possesses both energies. While the first keeps us alive, the second allows us to reach for our dreams and live a full life, filled with inspiration and motivation.

The Kabalists tell us that the energy of the shape of the letter *Cheit* represents a bridge (as in the Bridge Pose), which connects Earth to heaven, and us to the Divine. While the feet are grounded to the Earth, our hands are clasped or supporting the body, symbolically connecting us to all beings as part of the same body. When we are stable and in harmony between our inner heaven and our earthly attachment, the heart can open wide and create a space for the soul to express itself toward the ground and sky.

The sages explain that *Cheit* is also the symbol of a wheel of light that has no beginning and no end. It moves and turns for infinity, drawing the sacred light into all places and directions. When coming into the Wheel Pose, envision that you are this light carrying the unnatural energy in the most natural way, illuminating yourself and the space surrounding you. In the Wheel, as your heart lifts higher, a space is created underneath you and the Earth, representing the sacred space of light being drawn from your body into the ground. The space that surrounds your body is the infinite, where you can shine brightly and transform darkness into light.

Body

Poses:

Wheel Pose

Forearm Wheel

Reverse Table Top Pose

Wheel Pose

Create the kavana *(intention):*

Envision your heart as an altar being lifted into the sky to offer the light of your heart. This pose offers great energy both physically and mentally as it counteracts stress, depression, and anxiety.

Directions into the pose:

1. Lie on your back with the feet flat on the ground, and separate your feet hip-width apart.

2. Place your palms flat, next to the ears, fingertips pointing toward the shoulders.

3. Squeeze your elbows in so they are in line with your shoulder joints, and drop your shoulders away from your ears.

4. Exhale and tuck the tailbone.

5. As you inhale, press down through the soles of your feet and the palms of your hands, coming to the crown of the head. Most of your body weight should be supported by the hands.

6. Inhale, and expand your ribs.

7. Exhale, and connect to your midline, finding the beautiful balance through your breath, shining into your body.

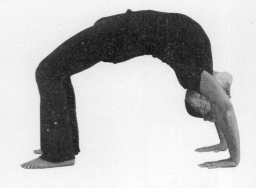

8. Draw your elbows in again so they are in line with your shoulders, and drop the shoulders down the back. This action is important to achieve before you lift up.

9. Exhale, then straighten your arms, and press your feet down to launch yourself into this incredible backward bend.

10. Open your heart and let your light shine.

11. Make sure your knees stay drawn in and hip-width apart, and that the toes are pointing forward and not out to the sides.

12. Let your neck be free, and breathe for five to ten breaths.

13. To come out, tuck your chin to your chest and slowly lower your hips to the ground. Gently extend the legs.

14. Close your eyes and feel the effects that this pose creates within the body.

Health and benefits:

- Opens the entire front and back of the body
- Stretches the muscles of the shoulders and backs of the legs
- Releases tension in the chest and the heart area
- Improves breathing and invites fresh oxygen into the body
- Can be a major emotional-releasing posture for people

Forearm Wheel

Create a kavana *intention:*

Envision your heart opening and shining as you lengthen your spine toward the Earth. This pose is an intense one that entails strength and a deep opening of the spine.

Directions into the pose:

1. From the Wheel Pose, bring the crown of your head to the ground.

2. Gently bring your forearms to the floor, one at a time, deepening your spine stretch.

3. Interlace your fingers behind your head, embracing your crown.

4. Draw your inner thighs toward your midline.

5. Press your feet and forearms to the Earth.

6. Lift your head off the Earth.

7. Feel elevated and yet connected to the Earth with no pressure on the top of your head.

Health and benefits:

*   Creates a deep opening in the chest and shoulders

*   Brings more flexibility and stretch to the spine

Reverse Table Top Pose

Create the kavana (*intention*):

See yourself as an altar holding energy ready to be offered from your heart. Reverse Table Top is a deep stretch to the upper body that opens the front of the body in an invigorating and energizing way to release fatigue and stress.

Directions into the pose:

1. Begin in a seated position with the legs straight out in front.

2. Place your hands on the floor about twelve inches behind your buttocks, fingers pointing toward the buttocks.

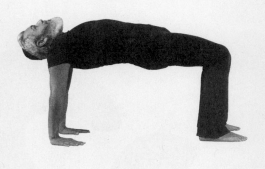

3. Inhale as you push down through your palms. With your feet separated hip-width, straighten your elbows and gently lift your hips up.

4. Drop your head back so that the crown of your head faces the back wall.

5. Breathe deeply and fully.

6. Hold the pose for five long breaths.

7. To come out, slowly lower your hips to the ground, and come into a passive forward bend.

Health and benefits:

•   Neutralizes forward bends by releasing the back and opening the front body

•   Stretches and tones the muscles in the front of the shoulders and the biceps

•   Creates tremendous release and expansion

CHAPTER 9

TET: Purpose

Pose: Crow Pose

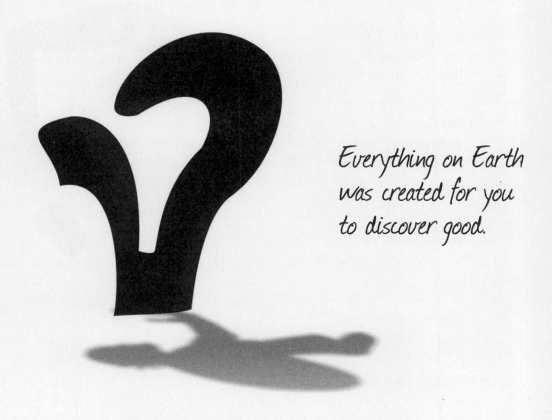

Everything on Earth was created for you to discover good.

The *Tet* corresponds to the English letter *T* and has a numerical value of 9.

Soul

Tet: Tet Afar Shenivra Mimeino Adam. "*Tet* ('good') is the soil from which man was created."

—Akivah

My teacher's (the Rebbe's) father-in-law, Rabbi Yosef Yitzchak Schneerson, shared the following incident that happened when he was a child. During the summer of 1896, young Yosef Yitzchak was taking a walk with his father through the countryside in Russia. The vegetation was almost ripe, and the grass rippled in a gentle breeze.

"Behold the Creator," his father said. "Every movement of each single seed of plant and blade of grass were included in the ancient thought, which causes each thing to be realized for a divine intention." As they strolled into a forest, the young boy meditated on what he had just learned from his father about divine providence.

While father and child walked together in the forest engrossed in deep meditation, the child plucked a leaf from a tree that he had passed without taking notice, and held it for a while in his hand. As the walk progressed into the forest, the child every so often tore off small pieces from the leaf and tossed them to the ground.

His father then said, "The mystic Arizal (Isaac, son of Solomon Luria Ashkenazi, 1534–1572) teaches that every leaf is a created being that has divine energy created with the intention of serving a purposeful role in creation." Then his father went on, "We were just discussing the subject of divine providence, and without awareness, you pulled a leaf off a tree, held it in your hand, played with it, tore it up into little pieces, and then scattered it. How can a person act with such unawareness? Whether it is a leaf or a person, each has a soul with a purpose to fulfill on Earth."

Most of us do not think in these terms. We are not in the habit of seeing the natural things of this world as possessing a soul and having a divine purpose. How many of us think of our life as more than what it is during this lifetime?

Generally speaking, each of us possesses at minimum the awareness to distinguish between what is good and bad, and to realize that we are responsible for some of our actions. We don't necessarily consider pulling a leaf off a tree as being a bad thing. But if the tearing of a leaf had no purpose, the leaf's life would have been cut short, and its soul would not have fulfilled its divine mission on Earth. If, however, the leaf was pulled off a branch in order to make medicine that could heal, or a tea that could be used to warm a cold body, then the leaf would have served a divine purpose on Earth by fulfilling a greater good. Everything on Earth is part of a greater whole, so when we do or do not do something, it affects a greater reality.

Purpose is something that we can cultivate, similar to what we do to the Earth when we prepare its soil to bear fruits. We irrigate the soil of life in order to eat, survive, and be satisfied. Intentions that are good and serve a positive purpose will be rooted into the divine intention that creates and sustains life in all things.

Your soul existed with a purpose long before this world was created and was consulted on how to best bring out the most good possible on Earth. Souls that come into this world experience many forms of evolution, transformation, and incarnation before entering a body. During each lifetime of your soul, a certain level of good is supposed to blossom through your purpose on Earth. Now is the most current adventure of the soul in your body. In the future, however, your purpose may be different. If we are in tune with our inner selves, then we will find this path with awareness. If we are not connected deeply, then divine fate will take us to our intended destination like a leaf in the wind being blown to a particular place without any discernible reason.

The Letter

The sages said about awareness, "Who is the wise man? The one who sees the birth of his intentions."[12] The letter *Tet* teaches us that our purpose on Earth is driven by our intentions.

The sages say that when selecting our intention, we need to be wise by envisioning the results that will flourish from our actions. When a thought comes to mind that may not be in line with the harmony we seek, its direction can be shifted at any time. The sages compare an intention to giving birth because it is something that is planted inside and grows, and when it is ready to be revealed, it is born into an action.

An intention gives birth to an experience. When from the outset the intention is positive, then the outcome will be positive. If the intention is negative, then this too will affect the experience.

Cultivating intention is something we learn to do as a baby. Parents' repetitive words and gestures cause a baby to react in a certain way. If they smile, then the baby will understand happiness and may smile back. If they show anger or speak harshly, the baby will react with sadness and fear. If the baby needs its diaper to be changed or is hungry, it will cry for attention. These baby moments are our original lessons about cause and effect that we learn in this lifetime.

Without realizing it, intention will be growing inside of us throughout our youth. As we move from childhood to where we are now, our life's challenges become more intense, and we learn how to channel intention more deeply. We become more responsible beings, we learn how to deepen our intentions and direct them into a certain purpose. Intention comes with maturity, and the more we learn how to savor life with all our senses, the closer we come to our purpose here on Earth in line with creating a world of good.

In the *Ethics of the Fathers*, it is said that Judah the Prince used to say: "What is above you is because of you."[13] The connection between cause and effect is something that goes beyond our physical realm. Everything on Earth, and each of us, is rooted into a higher movement that governs our planet and directs us into our purpose. Our thoughts, words, and actions will affect this spiritual movement that hovers over us. Our intentions will influence the way we receive from the source of life and live our purpose on Earth.

If the intention is positive, then you reveal light in your actions. If the intention is negative, then this can conceal light and cause negative things to happen. Each action has its consequences. The action we experience will always be driven by an accumulation of previous intentions gathered together, which affect the flow of your life. Thoughts become part of your personality, and what you see with your eyes, hear with your ears, smell with your nose, and eat with your mouth will enter into you and become a part of you.

Because your soul is rooted in the Creator's soul, it has been carrying the very same light since creation. Depending on your incarnation and purpose in each lifetime, your soul will illuminate in a certain way, differently from the past. All of us, except for a few new souls, have lived many lives. The advantage of having an "old soul" is that the soul returns to Earth in order to complete or correct a certain pattern of the past. Rarely will a new soul descend. The sages say that a new soul comes down only when there is to be something new that the world has never seen before, something necessary for the healing of Earth and humankind.

During the lifetime of the body and soul, there is a purpose the body and soul must fulfill together. Each time we create a good intention, it awakens the original good your soul consented to prior to Creation and inspires good deeds to follow, which in turn can lead to future positivity. A negative intention, on the other hand, will deviate from the original good your soul agreed to and experienced, and may cause negativity.

Physical life ceases when the purpose is attained. The soul, after spending some time in the eternal light, comes back to Earth in another form of life with a new purpose to fulfill.

Breath: Energetic Shape and Intention

The kavanas *of the Tet are all forms of positive intentions that bring change, such as passion, trust, hope, love, compassion, and understanding of your body—the awareness of your being now rooted, yet lifted and connected to all life.*

The *Tet* is the Crow Pose, which is one of the first balancing arm poses we learn in yoga. This pose stretches the upper back and strengthens the arms, wrists, and abdominal muscles. The inhale in the Crow is at the pressing down of the hands and lengthening of the spine as the heart opens inward. The inhale is also at the gathering of the upper body, as you draw into the navel and squeeze the knees together. The exhale is the strengthening of your upper arms, forearms, and wrists. The exhale is also the settling of the body behind the arms, as the hands press down to the Earth. It is also the strengthening into the abdominals and torso.

The Side Crow Pose works our strength and focus. The inhale is at the lengthening of the spine, the exhale at the twisting. The inhale is also at the lifting of the body and the exhale at the pressing down of the hands upon the Earth. The shape of the letter *Tet* is similar to an inverted container. This pose reminds us to view our body as a container that carries a purpose. When you press down on your hands, imagine that you are opening your heart wide. Within us exists this light of good, and we should channel it into our lives. When coming into the Crow Pose or Side Crow, imagine that you are lifting yourself higher to enjoy the blessings surrounding you. The *Tet*, lifted above the Earth, represents the elevation of the body.

The *Tet* can also be shaped as the Bridge Pose with the palms pressed to the Earth, supporting the hips or with the fingers clasped. The Bridge Pose shows us that we can elevate the heart as we bring the hips higher, and yet remain connected to the Earth with our arms, fingers, and feet. In the Bridge Pose, the inhale is the pressing of the feet to the Earth and the lifting of the hips. It is also the lengthening of the tailbone and its extension from the pelvis through the knees. The exhale is at the supporting of the hips or clasping of the hands under you, as the shoulder blades connect to each other. It is at the pressing of the feet before you inhale to lift the body.

The intention of the *Tet* is to see the potential good in all areas and cultivate in your heart this feeling of good, remembering that this good already exists within, and all we need to do is move inward.

Body

Poses:

Crow Pose

Side Crow Pose

Bridge Pose

Crow Pose

Create the kavana (*intention*):

You are an elevated being that draws from the Earth into the dynamic above you. In this pose, you strengthen your core, arms, and wrists, as you find balance and concentration.

Directions into the pose:

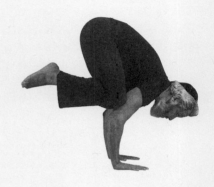

1. From a squat position, place your hands in front of your feet, flat on the ground and shoulder-width apart.

2. Let your elbows bend and the knees drop onto the triceps or into the armpits.

3. Lean forward and lower your head and chest toward the ground.

4. Lift your heels, come onto the tips of your toes, and lift your tailbone high toward the sky.

5. Contract your abdomen in and up toward the spine, and squeeze your elbows into your torso, pushing your knees into your arms while beginning to transfer your weight forward onto your palms.

6. Set your gaze a few inches ahead of your hands.

7. Finally, lift one foot off the ground and then the other. Bring the big toes together.

8. Breathe deeply and evenly, and attempt to balance for thirty seconds.

Health and benefits:

- Tones and strengthens the whole body
- Improves the ability to deal with frustration and fear

Side Crow Pose

Create the kavana (*intention*):

Imagine that by lifting your body, you are raising your level of awareness. This pose works your core and arm strength and builds concentration.

Directions into the pose:

1. Come into a squat with your knees together and feet pressed together, heels up.

2. Bring your hands together to your heart.

3. On an exhale, twist your torso to the right, lift your hips, and place your hands flat on the ground to your right; keep your arms shoulder-width apart.

4. Spread your fingers apart wide and distribute your weight evenly into both hands.

5. Keep your elbows slightly bent as you start to move your body forward.

6. Start leaning on your upper arms.

7. Your outer right hip should rest on the back of your right upper arm, while your right knee should be against the back of your left upper arm.

8. Keep your knees together.

9. Slowly press down through your right hip and lift your feet up.

10. Maintain the feet and legs parallel to the floor; your arms can lengthen and straighten when you are ready.

11. Gaze forward toward the horizon. Return your feet to the floor. Repeat on the other side.

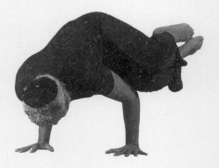

Health and benefits:

- Strengthens the arms, shoulders, wrists, abdominal muscles, and spine

- Increases awareness and self-confidence

Bridge Pose

Create the kavana (*intention*):

Your heart is lifted higher as you draw energy from the Earth into the dynamic above you. This pose builds your core and lower body strength, lengthens and strengthens the spine, and energizes the body as you find balance and focus.

Directions into the pose:

1. Lie on your back and place your feet flat on the ground, hip-width apart.

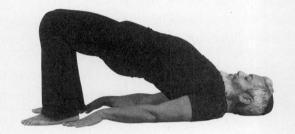

2. Stack your knees over your heels. The distance of your feet from your hips is approximately where the tip of your middle finger grazes the backs of your heels.

3. Inhale to scoop your tailbone under and lift your hips up high, resting on your shoulders.

4. Roll your right shoulder under and then your left, and press your palms flat into the ground. (Alternatively, clasp your hands a together to interlock your fingers.)

5. Keep pressing down equally through both feet and your upper arms and palms.

6. Maintain the knees hip-width apart but begin to spin your inner thighs toward the ground.

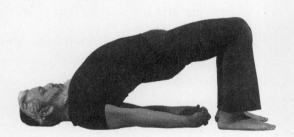

7. Set your gaze to the tip of your nose.

8. On your inhalation, feel the rib cage and chest expand.

9. On your exhalation, push firmly through your feet and palms as you lift your hips up high. Stay here for several breaths.

Health and benefits:

- Opens the chest and the abdominal wall
- Stimulates the thyroid and improves digestion
- Helps relieve mild depression
- Tones the buttocks, thighs, and lower back
- Creates a deeper connection to breathing

CHAPTER 10

YUD: Hide-and-Seek

Pose: Forward Bend

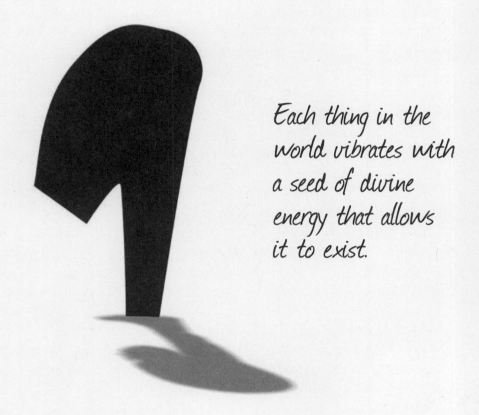

Each thing in the world vibrates with a seed of divine energy that allows it to exist.

The *Yud* corresponds to the English letters *I* and *Y* and has a numerical value of 10.

Soul

Yud: Yodu Al Kol Ma'asecha Bechol Yom. "Through *Yud* (a seed) all of creation will know you."

—Akivah

One Friday afternoon, I managed to get home earlier than usual for the start of *shabbat* (the Saturday day of rest), which begins at sunset. As I sat on a cushion in my living room, I attempted to close my eyes and look inward, to empty my busy mind by meditating into silence. Suddenly, my children came downstairs and started playing a loud game of hide-and-seek. My mind could not resist their lively game, and so instead of meditating inwardly, I kept my eyes open and watched the kids run and play.

Like many children, my kids love playing this game. Geoulah, my oldest daughter, was the first one to be the seeker on this occasion. While the others ran frantically all over the house, she covered her face with a pillow and counted to sixty. I heard her whisper, "fifty-eight, fifty-nine, sixty," and the hunt began. Tanya, who was then only three years old, hid underneath the dining room table that was covered with a white tablecloth in honor of the *shabbat*. Because she could not see anyone, she imagined that no one could see her either, but her giggling gave her away, and she was the first to be found.

In a frenzied chase, Geoulah started searching every room of the house for her siblings. This time they outdid themselves—I was quite impressed by how well they hid. They knew of places that I had never thought of. Maayan, my second oldest daughter, took cover behind a pile of laundry, and my son Shamai, the eldest, concealed himself in the bottom of the winter closet. But my son Tsem's hiding place was a mystery. At first Geoulah was frustrated, but suddenly she heard the laundry basket fall on the ground and caught Maayan. Geoulah then headed for the winter closet. She opened the door and looked inside, but saw nothing. Then a soft sound came from the recesses of the closet and, sure enough, Shamai was discovered. Only Tsem had yet to be found.

He had hidden so well that at this point, all the kids were looking for him. I was actually a bit concerned. Finally, after the excitement about the game had waned, the kids decided that it was over, and each went on to do their own thing. Everyone disappeared, and the house was suddenly quiet again. I could now close my eyes and focus on my breath, but I wondered, *Where is Tsem?* He finally came running out of his hiding place, to discover that the game was over without him ever being caught. Now he was doing the searching, looking for where everyone had gone. He may have won the game, but I could see from the look on his face that he did not feel as though he was a winner because he was never found and was not as joyful as he would have been had he been caught.

I thought to myself, *Did Tsem really win the game? Or did he lose?* This thought caused me to meditate about the game of hide-and-seek we often play with ourselves. Isn't it true that sometimes we try to hide? How often do we hide from our friends, from our family, and even from ourselves? We find very creative ways to do this—disappearing behind mental and emotional shields and between layers of undertakings. Sometimes we find refuge somewhere in the past or in a dream of a beautiful future, just to not have to be in the present.

The Hassidic teachings speak of two types of concealment: a "concealment," and a "concealment within a concealment." The first type of concealment is the Creator hiding behind the layers of nature, making it seem as though everything is happening automatically by days, months, years, and seasons.

The second level—concealment within a concealment—is similar to the game of hide-and-seek, where the Creator purposely hides himself in order to arouse within us a desire to find him and be deeply connected. At this stage, we find the Creator by exerting efforts to refine our personality, by improving our character, and by looking deeply within ourselves.

The Letter

The dot of the *Yud* carries both concealments. While within it is contained all of life, it is also the seed that brings change and transformation.

The mystics describe the Creator as hiding in the small folded shape of the letter *Yud.* Similar to a seed planted in the ground carrying the entire length, width, and dimension of the tree, the *Yud* carries within it the infinite seed of energy that would bring life to Earth. For a seed to grow into a fruit-bearing tree, it must be nurtured with water, sunlight, air, and the nutrients of the Earth. To blossom, the world also requires a heart to feel warmth, love, and compassion, and air to breathe life in harmony. It needs water to nourish its growth, passions, and dreams, and an Earth from where it can stand rooted and build a space of movement and activity.

The Creator hides himself from us so well that it can be hard to believe that he exists. Although it may feel as though it is we who are running the world, the Creator is here, making everything happen. If you ask exactly where the Creator is, the answer will never be clear. It's not that the Creator is nowhere, but there is nowhere that he is not. In reality, the Creator is everywhere. Having ears does not mean we will automatically hear the eternal being, although if we listen carefully, we can notice him making some noise. When there is thunder or lightning, our reaction is to say that it's nature reacting to the collision of clouds. When an earthquake occurs somewhere in the world, we explain it as a natural catastrophe. But beyond the clouds and winds of life, and Mother Nature, is the Creator acting in our world. Having eyes does not mean that we will necessarily see the Creator. We may recognize sounds, signs, and wonders of life, but this does not mean that we will hear, see, and feel the Creator in the way we do the things and people around us. Rather, the hearing, seeing, and feeling come from our internal senses connected to our soul. We cannot expect to experience the Creator in the same way that we do anything physical in the world. To connect with the Creator, we need to reach beyond all layers until there are none left, not even a thought.

Hiddenness is what makes the Creator beyond us, mysterious, and complex. The Creator would not be the infinite force of life if he were not somewhat detached from all of existence. As Hasidic master the Kotzker Rebbe once said, "I would not want to worship a God whose every way of being I could understand."

He is beyond our understanding of reality. He is not what we think he is, and yet he is very close to each of us. The Creator chooses to hide himself so we learn to see and feel him through awareness. Perhaps this is the reason why the Creator plays with us a game of hide-and-seek—so we come to know him on our own terms and discover that he is everything and everywhere in our lives. The Creator conceals himself so we remember him in our joy, in our sadness, and in every breath we take.

Breath: Energetic Shape and Intention

The kavanas of the Yud are feelings of humility, selflessness, introversion, and soulfulness. The intention is also to open the heart to love, compassion, passion, and understanding.

In the Child Pose, the inhale is at the extension of the spine while creating space in your body. The inhale is also the lifting of the heart, as you take in the energy surrounding you and connect to a higher energy above you. The exhale is the folding of the body to the Earth and the drawing of the heart into the depths of yourself. It is the melting of the body and the settling of the heart into the ground as you plant rays of light that will shine. It is deeply rooting in order to shine higher and begin your journey.

Shiva Rea, creator of Prana Vinyasa, calls this pose the Wisdom Pose: "It is the wisdom of knowing when to relax and come back to yourself. It is the wisdom of knowing when you need to take a break for your body."[14] I love this name, as it represents the *Yud*, which carries the seed of wisdom of the Creator within its petite shape.

There are variations and modifications you can take in the Child Pose and the Forward Bend Pose. In the Child Pose, you can have your arms resting at your sides with the palms facing upward and your forehead resting on the floor. Alternatively, another variation is for the arms to be stretched above the head in a shoulder flexion.

For the lower body, a variation can include opening the knees to allow the belly to be drawn to the floor, and you can envision the fire within you connecting to the Earth. Your forehead can rest on your hands, stacked and with your head turned to one side. Your arms can be by the sides of your body or holding onto your heels.

In the Forward Bend, you can hold your elbows or grab your legs or heels as a way of connecting deeper to yourself.

The *Yud* is the smallest Hebrew letter, and its shape is assumed by folding oneself to the ground, such as in the Child Pose or the Melting Heart Pose, where the front of the body is melted into the Earth. It is also shaped while standing in the Forward Bend, where the upper body is lengthened downward and the heart draws into the thighs while the crown of the head reaches for the Earth. The Squat Pose can also be the shape of the *Yud* as it is a grounding one that helps us tap into a downward-flowing energy and is great for bringing a sense of calm.

The *Yud* shapes our body like a seed folded inward as a reminder that everything exists inside of us. When we look inward with humility, we see from the perspective of the Creator all of life, including the Earth, air, sun, and water, all constantly nourishing our existence.

Body

Poses:

Rag Doll and Forward Bend

Squat Pose

Wide-Knees Child Pose with Arms Outstretched

Melting Heart Pose

Rag Doll and Forward Bend

Create the kavana (*intention*):

Envision your heart softly hanging toward the Earth and releasing its energy. This gentle variation of a standing Forward Bend relaxes the body and mind, while actively stretching the whole back of the body.

Directions into the pose:

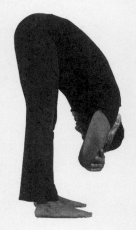

1. Begin in Downward Dog.

2. Soften the hamstrings (the backs of your legs) and slowly walk your feet forward to rest between your hands.

3. Inhale as you lengthen the spine, exhale, and then fold your torso forward and grab your elbows.

4. Let your head hang heavy and your spine lengthen toward the ground.

5. You can sway from side to side or nod the head yes and no to release the neck.

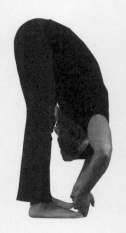

6. Breathe deeply into the sides of the body and let the ribs expand with your breath.

7. To go deeper in the pose, grab the insides of your big toes.

8. Inhale as you energetically pull your big toes down and exhale as you bend over; then bend your elbows and roll your shoulders away from your ears.

9. Continue to work opposing movements as you push your feet into the ground: lift your tailbone up to the ceiling and lengthen your heart toward the ground.

10. Remain for five breaths. You can release your hands next to your feet and stay a few breaths longer.

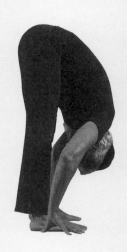

Health and benefits:

- Lengthens the spine and the backs of the legs
- Relaxes the neck and encourages fresh blood flow to the brain
- Stimulates and "rinses" the organs and the belly, including the digestive system
- Brings a sense of harmony to the brain chemistry

Squat Pose

Create the kavana (*intention*):

As you ground yourself, think of opening your heart energy into the space of your hips. The Squat Pose, also known as Garland Pose, has the effect of grounding, or connecting into a downward flow of energy that brings calmness.

Directions into the pose:

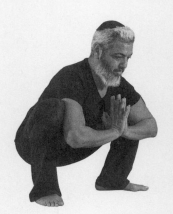

1. Begin in Mountain Pose, with your feet a bit wider than hip-width apart.

2. Inhale, pivot your feet out, and spread your toes.

3. Exhale, bend your knees, and lower your hips below your knees, close to the Earth.

4. Inhale, and bring your hands together to your heart, your elbows inside your knees.

5. Exhale, and gently press your elbows into your knees to open your hips.

6. Inhale, lift your heart forward toward the sky, and lengthen into your spine and lower back.

7. Remain for thirty seconds to one minute.

8. To come out of the pose, either press your feet down into a standing position or softly sit back onto your buttocks.

Health and benefits:

- Releases the lower back
- Opens the hips
- Strengthens the ankles

Wide-Knees Child Pose with Arms Outstretched

Create the kavana *(intention):*

Your body is the shell that carries your soul, the seed of life that brings growth. Let your body melt down to the Earth as you bring awareness to the energy below you.

Directions into the pose:

1. Come onto your hands and knees.

2. Inhale, bring your big toes together, and separate your knees mat-width apart.

3. Exhale, and allow your belly to draw down into the Earth.

4. Let the weight of your hips sink toward your heels.

5. Inhale, and extend your arms straight out in front of you, palms facing the ground.

6. Exhale, and let everything relax as you connect to your body and your breathing.

7. Let your breath soothe and center you.

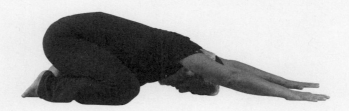

Health and benefits:

- Restores the heart rate and calms the nervous system
- Deeply restores the entire body

Melting Heart Pose

Create the kavana *(intention):*

Envision yourself planting your heart into the Earth as if you were planting a seed. This posture allows the heart to melt toward the Earth while stretching the spine in both directions.

Directions into the pose:

1. From Child Pose, softly bring your fingers out in front of you. Gently lower your chest and forehead down so your forehead is resting on the Earth.

2. Your hips should be over your knees and your arms shoulder-distance apart.

3. Softly press your palms downward as you lift your elbows up.

4. As your hips reach toward the sky, draw your shoulder blades down your back.

5. Keep your neck soft and lengthen your spine.

6. Maintain a relaxed and calm breath.

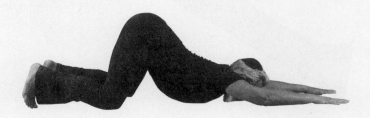

Health and benefits:

• Opens the heart

• Stretches the spine, upper back, shoulders, and arms

• Relieves stress and anxiety

CHAPTER 11

KHAF: Power

Pose: Downward Dog

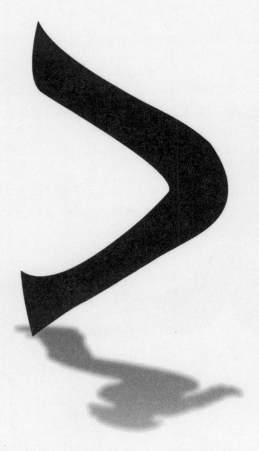

Power is embracing the hidden energy that comes from your essence.

The *Khaf* corresponds to the English letter *K* and has a numerical value of 20.

Soul

Khaf: Kevod Adonai Ala-ich Zarach. "The glory of the Creator radiates in me."

—Akivah

The sages relate *(midrash)* that when the Earth was created and the birds came into existence, they were initially given the art of singing melodies. The Creator had also made wings upon their backs, which at first served no purpose except for being a heavy burden. The birds complained to the Creator that although they were happy to sing, still they had to drag these heavy useless wings on their feeble bodies. The Creator, amused by their protest, said to the feathered creatures, "I see justice in your concern. Let us wait a week, and if you are still unhappy, I shall remove from you these heavy wings." The birds left very confident that they had well pleaded their case. A day later, a strange thing happened. They suddenly began to feel a wind lifting them above the Earth, and after a few days, they were flying high up in the sky. The following week, the birds appeared again before the Creator, humbled. "Master of the universe, how did we doubt your eternal wisdom? The wings that we thought were useless, we will now use them to sing to you for allowing us to soar high into heaven and be close to you."

Prior to your soul's descent on Earth, it was given unique powers—*kochos* (discussed in more detail in chapter 7), the meaning of the letter *Khaf*—with which to be transformed. The soul, however, was told neither how to go about finding these powers nor which intentions—*kavana*, another meaning of the *Khaf*—to have in order to soar high and freely engage in the human experience as it discovers life on its own.

Your soul did not simply come to Earth because your parents decided to have you. You came because the Creator desired that you exist. Since the beginning of time, the world has been eagerly waiting for your soul to arrive and fulfill its particular role. A soul does not only come into a body to complete or correct a past life. It also comes in order to offer its own special light that has never existed before. Without your soul, creation could never be complete. Neither the Earth nor the sky, with all its wonders and awesomeness, would be the same had your soul not been chosen to do its part on Earth.

Your soul is similar to a field that can blossom if cultivated. Just as a seed, for your soul to grow, it needs a heart (sun) to shine, mind (water) to flow, and oxygen (air) to breathe. The power, *koach* (pronounced "ko-ach"), of the soul is that it is the spiritual soil where seeds of *kavana*, "intentions," are cultivated. We can begin our life cultivating one way and change it several times before finding the soil of our heart's desires where our hidden powers can be discovered.

The Baal Shem Tov, a nineteenth century mystic known as the founder of the Hasidic movement, made the following observation concerning the soil of your soul:

> The Earth is filled with treasures, precious metals, and gemstones, hidden deep in the ground. To find them you must dig, and when you discover them, you have to clear away the dirt and impurities. Then they must be refined, brightened, and worked on. So too each of us possesses powers and strength that are often hidden and buried deep inside the soul. The more we irrigate this spiritual soil of the soul, the further we will reach into our hidden powers, which leads to discovering our role on Earth.[15]

To savor the soul's embrace of the human experience, sometimes we need to look from outside ourselves and observe. What do you see? Compassion? Love? Beauty? Are you hard and judgmental? Are you understanding and patient?

My teacher, the Rebbe, would often compare such a person to a lamplighter, whose occupation is to stand on the outside in order to illuminate darkness. Internally, this happens when we start to dig deeper into our inner terrain, slowly stripping away layers of accumulated fears, ego, and limitations that hide our precious jewels—the intentions of our soul. While the *koach*, the hidden treasure of your potential, is symbolized by the outer layer of your soul, *kavana*, "inner feelings," is the inner layer of your soul. *Kavana*, say the mystics, is cultivated either in the soil of the mind or in the Earth of the heart. When we have an intention in the mind, we have a vision of what we wish to see happen. This vision empowers us to be more focused and determined to realize what we see. When the *kavana* is grown in the heart, what is produced is emotions that, when channeled, bring out passion and deep feelings we desire to experience. We awaken love, compassion, forgiveness, and understanding. Whether the intention is from the mind or from the heart, both work together to bring out the greatest intention. One can view the heart being below the mind as a way of lifting its warm flames into our focus and concentration in the brain (which can be cold and calculating) with more clarity and depth.

The soul has many dwellings. Depending on the powers it must grow into, it will be given the skills to fulfill its role. A soul may dwell in the body of a healer who finds cures to ailments, or in a dreamer who inspires people, or in a leader who brings hope to a changing world, or in a mother destined to raise a beautiful family, founded on love, affection, and sincerity. Your role may be to bring joy, to be a muse, to teach, or to influence people with the talents you have been blessed with.

The journey of the soul is similar to a highway. It can take us in a certain direction but also include roads and exits that lead to other cities and towns; so too our life journey may take us on several roads as we travel to our specific destination. Have the side roads taken us off the course of our path? Not necessarily. When we travel long distances on a major highway, we often stop to get some fuel, food, and rest so we can ultimately reach our destination. The universe also causes us to interrupt our journeys, not to throw us off the road of our focus, but to slow us down in order to be present, to heal what needs to be cured, to improve what requires amelioration, or to reach out to someone on the way who needs a helping hand.

The Letter

The *Khaf* teaches us that to be powerful is to be humble. The letter is powerful because it is grounding, heartfelt, and connective, like the Downward Dog Pose. It is humble because its shape is that of bowing down. Power is often judged according to one's money, influence, and status in society. The letter *Khaf* teaches us that true power must be viewed from one's inner power. People with such power are devoid of ego, knowing that any talent they have been blessed with is a gift from heaven. They realize that the Creator could have given this power to anyone else but chose them instead. They are not concerned with superficial or materialistic desires. Instead, they live simply and humbly. They do not look for control or domination. Rather, they are openhearted and spiritual. They see a light in all people. For such a powerful person, it is clear that every person, no matter what their status is in society, has a soul directly connected to the Creator. For such a person, it does not make a difference whether you are rich, poor, or famous. A powerful person sees each body as a vessel carrying light to brighten the world and beautify its path on Earth.

The universe does not judge us for which occupation we assume in our lifetime, but for how much of our soul was invested in what we did. The sages of *The Talmud* say that when the soul returns back to the Creator, it is asked four questions: Did you labor with faith? Did you cultivate and irrigate? Did you learn? Did you have hopes and dreams?[16]

If we approach life with awareness, then we will see where the bigger road takes us and navigate our sojourns with more direction. Our "stops" in life are not interruptions but a continuous movement into the bigger picture of our personal lives.

To be a powerful person is to be grateful for the opportunities of life; to give expression to your soul as you fulfill your part on Earth; and to cultivate compassion, understanding, and love in your heart to share with others regardless of who they are.

Breath: Energetic Shape and Intention

The kavanas of the Khaf are feelings of rootedness and the opening of your heart to feelings of love, compassion, and soulfulness. While the intention is to plant your heart into the Earth in such poses as Downward Dog and Plank Pose, the intention in the Upward Facing Dog Pose is to open the heart upward toward the sky with powerful feelings inside you.

In the Downward Dog Pose, the inhale is at the extension of the upper body, while placing the hands and fingers on the Earth, open like stars. The inhale is also the lifting of the heart, as you coil in the energy from the Earth through the hands and feet. The exhale is the rooting down into the Earth and the drawing of the heart into the depths of yourself. It is the melting of the upper body downward and the settling of the heart toward the ground as you plant rays of light that will shine through your fingers.

The *Khaf* is a bowing-down posture that physically relates to our submissiveness and humility toward a greater power. The Downward Dog, Plank, Upward Facing Dog, and Cobra are poses important to the *Khaf*, and relate to the Salutations, which are often practiced prior to doing a series of poses.

Khaf is also the Hebrew word for the palms of the hands, which teaches us that while doing any of these posture variations, the light of your soul emanates through the fingers into the Earth. Particularly, when coming into the Downward Dog Pose, the hands should be rooted and the fingers spread evenly as shining stars. Also, by bending and pressing the hands down and away from the Earth, the hips are elevated to the sky while the bottom of the spine lengthens upward for the heart to be above the head.

All poses of the *Khaf* form the basis of the Salutations, which are opportunities to irrigate deeply into the wisdom of the body by revealing more from a warm heart, to create intentions (*kavana*) that will inspire our flow.

In the Downward Dog Pose, the intention is to honor life and its source as we open from the inside out with the heart above the mind. The Plank Pose's intention is to lengthen the body horizontally from the heels to the top of the head as if drawing a line of energy. In the Upward Facing Dog Pose, the intention is to hover horizontally over the Earth and yet keep the heart and mind above the body in order to connect to the energy above us.

In the Cobra Pose, the inhale is at the lifting of the heart from the Earth while the exhale is as you lengthen your spine and keep connected to the energy underneath you.

Body

Poses:

Downward Dog Pose

Plank Pose

Upward Facing Dog Pose

Cobra Pose

Downward Dog Pose

Create the kavana (*intention*):

Plant your heart toward the Earth so that everything positive inside of you grows deeply throughout your body. Downward Dog is considered a mild inversion because the heart is above the head. It strengthens and stretches the entire body and is essential to the Salutations, or as a connecting movement between postures.

Directions into the pose:

1. Begin in a table-top position with your hands and knees on the Earth.

2. Bring your wrists under your shoulders and your knees under your hips.

3. Spread your fingers wide and press down through your palms.

4. Allow your body weight to be distributed evenly through the hands.

5. Tuck your toes under and lift your knees above the Earth.

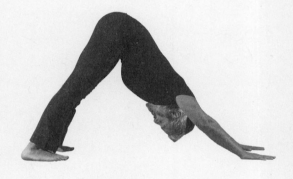

6. Lift your hips toward the ceiling and press your sitting bones back.

7. Bring your thighs back as you start to straighten your legs.

8. Spiral the tops of the thighs inward and keep the outer thighs firm as you draw the upper thighs slightly inward.

9. Keep pressing away from the ground through the palms of your hands as you lengthen the tailbone and lift from your pelvis.

10. Breathe fully and freely throughout your back.

11. Firm your arms and draw your shoulder blades to your upper back ribs.

12. Visualize your hips and thighs being drawn backward toward your essence above you.

Health and benefits:

- Calms the brain, and relieves stress and mild depression
- Energizes the entire body
- Improves digestion and back pain
- Helps relieve symptoms of menopause, headaches, insomnia, and fatigue

Plank Pose

Create the kavana (*intention*):

Envision lengthening your heart horizontally as you extend energy to the crown of your head and to the soles of your feet. Plank is a foundational pose that asks you to gather yourself together powerfully, similar to a wooden plank, as you embrace strength for the practice.

Directions into the pose:

1. Come onto your hands and knees.

2. Bring your wrists directly under your shoulders.

3. Spread your fingers apart evenly and press down through your hands and forearms.

4. Keep your chest lifted, and lengthen the back of your neck as you look to the Earth.

5. Draw your abdominal muscles to your spine and breathe deeper.

6. Scoop your toes under and energetically press your feet back.

7. Create a horizontal line between your heels and the top of your head.

8. Expand your shoulder blades and collarbones.

9. A modification of the Plank Pose is to place your knees on the Earth while holding the pose for at least five breaths.

10. To go into low plank pose, hug your elbows in and lower your body parallel to the floor. Your shoulders and elbows should be at the same height.

11. Stay a few breaths, deeply connecting with your inner strength before releasing to lie fully on the floor.

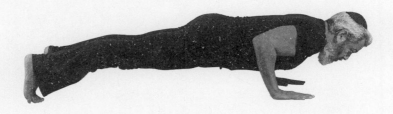

Health and benefits:

- Tones the core muscles, including the chest, abdomen, and lower back
- Strengthens the arms, wrists, and shoulders, as well as the muscles supporting the spine

Upward Facing Dog Pose

Create the kavana (*intention*):

Elevate your heart from the Earth so the cultivations you do within grow deeply throughout your body. The Upward Facing Dog, a common pose in a flow sequence, is a strong pose that vitalizes the upper body and stretches the chest and abdomen.

Directions into the pose:

1. From a low push-up, press your hands down and scoop the belly in and up.

2. Push your chest forward and up through your hands.

3. Push the bottoms of the feet back. Squeeze your buttocks to engage your thighs.

4. Move your shoulders back and down, and lift the chest high.

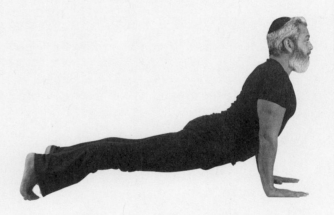

Health and benefits:

- Stretches the entire front of the torso

- Opens the chest and the heart center

- Opens the shoulders and tones the muscles of the arms

Cobra Pose

Create the kavana (*intention*):

Elevate your heart from the Earth and yet remain close to the Earth as you begin to reveal the fruits within your body. The Cobra Pose is a good backbend for beginners and a great way to open the heart while strengthening the spine and making it more flexible.

Directions into the pose:

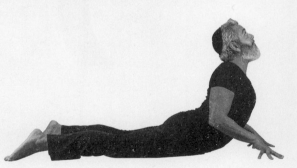

1. Lie on your belly.

2. Position your big toes to touch; heels should be a few inches apart.

3. Place your palms down at the level of your chest.

4. Squeeze your elbows close to the torso and draw the shoulder blades toward your waist, drawing them in toward one another.

5. Inhale as you peel your chest from the ground while continuing to push actively through the tops of your feet.

6. Keep your chin facing the ground as you work to keep your neck in line with your spine.

7. Breathe into your lower back and visualize it lifting and lengthening.

8. Stay for five breaths and then release. You can deepen the pose by lifting from your fingertips.

9. Rest for a few breaths, inviting complete relaxation into the body.

Health and benefits:

- Strengthens the lower back and the muscles between the shoulder blades
- Improves posture
- Stretches the abdomen and chest
- Relieves lower back pain

CHAPTER 12

LAMED: Learning and Teaching
Pose: Upward Salute

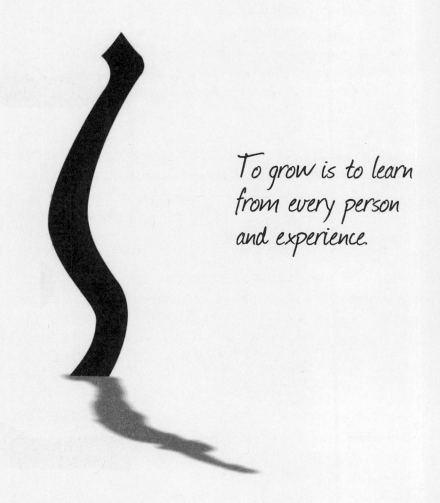

To grow is to learn from every person and experience.

The *Lamed* corresponds to the English letter *L* and has a numerical value of 30.

Soul

Lamed: Lev Mevin Da'at. "The heart is understanding."

—Akivah

The Talmud relates that the sage Rabbah was a spectacular *Lamed,* the Hebrew word for "teacher" and the name of the tallest Hebrew letter. Rabbah knew how to get his students' attention. He would often begin teaching his students with jokes and humor to open their senses, loosen them up, and make them laugh. Once everyone was present and comfortable, he would then begin his teaching, using the joke as the starting point to learning great lessons of life. The sages of *The Talmud* raved about his method, and explained that a teacher should learn from Rabbah, who could literally "open his students" before entering into their hearts and minds to share a deep teaching.

The Letter

The *Lamed* is the tallest letter, as it reaches above all the sacred shapes and symbolizes a transmission from above to below. This handing-over must be from the heart, *lev,* also a symbol of the *Lamed.* In its shape, the heart of the letter *Lamed* is situated right above the point from where the lower part of the letter begins to draw down. The heart of the letter *Lamed* extends beyond its body to tell us that a teacher should offer their lessons from the wisdom and voice of their heart.

I was privileged to have such a teacher who taught in a special way. Rabbi Shlomo Benarosch, known to us as Rebi, was my Torah teacher from grade one to grade six. In grade one, he taught me how to read the Torah and write in Hebrew. Later on, I learned from him how to read Aramaic so I could understand the language of *The Babylonian Talmud* (500 CE). He was down-to-earth and one of the best teachers I ever had. I remember the lessons I learned from him when I was six years old more vividly than things I learned later in life. That is because he gave so much of himself that even today I can still hear his voice in my heart.

Although he was old enough to be my grandfather, he was young at heart, funny, caring, and understanding. He was a tall man with a long white beard that reminded me of Charlton Heston in the movie *The Ten Commandments.* He was charismatic and had a powerful voice that could be heard beyond the walls of the classroom, especially when he sang chants of the ancestors. He knew how to get the class interested in learning. He would tell us jokes and stories and let us have extra time for recess if we behaved. Sometimes, to keep our attention, he played a game of Simon Says, where each of us took turns being Simon. Of course, we had to be respectful and not make fun of Rebi. Once, it was my turn, and that day I was in a funny mood. I said to the rabbi, "Simon says do Elvis Presley." The classroom was all giggles as the students looked to see his reaction. I was known to be a big Elvis fan, but no one knew that Rebi was an even bigger fan than me. He suddenly grabbed his long ruler, held it in his arms like a guitar and started shaking his left leg, swinging it back and forth, and with his deep voice sang "Blue Suede Shoes."

Rebi connected with us by coming to our level. He got through to me because he taught with love. Love is like *lev*, the Hebrew word for "heart," spelled with a *Lamed*. Love is the most essential ingredient in any relationship because it opens us to gratitude, sensitivity, compassion, and much more. Without a heart, love can never be expressed.

I am forever Rebi's student, *lomed*, which is another way of pronouncing *Lamed*, for the things he taught me have stayed with me. The reason why the letter *Lamed* also has the meaning of "student" *(lomed)* is to tell us that the goal of a teacher is not just to transmit information but also to teach in a way that the student can apply the teachings. For this to happen, a teacher needs to live by their teachings.

Ultimately, we want our children and students to stand on their own feet and think, feel, and figure things out independent of our influence. When our students internalize the wisdom we impart, in turn they become teachers, having the role of living and sharing the knowledge they received to their own children and students of life.

Ideally, a teacher should have a positive personality where they can help us see the greater good and want to make a difference in the world. Rebi was also a talented painter known in the community for making incredible artwork that depicted stories of the Bible. Every one of his paintings told a story. You could tell that Rebi painted with great emotion. I, too, loved to draw, and Rebi always took the time to look at my work and help me enhance my art. At the age of twelve, I met with him each Sunday for my bar mitzvah lessons, over the course of an entire year. After almost every session, we would also spend time drawing together so I could see how he did it. It was always amazing to see Rebi at work. He was blind in one eye, so he always tilted his head to the left in order to see better from his good eye. He had big strong hands. Still, he held a pencil so gracefully and would very softly make contact of the pencil to the paper. He would say to me, "God gave us two eyes, one that looks inward, and the other that sees outward. God gave me one eye that sees both ways!"

A teacher should be humble. With humility and pride, Rebi showed me how to tap into my creativity, to see from deep within. How to handle a sketching pad, to be confident when holding a pencil in my hand, and to always be gentle with each stroke I make. He would say to me, "The world came from nothing. You see this nothingness (pointing at the empty sheet of paper); now create something beautiful."

From the simple teachings of Rebi, I have learned to see myself not as the origin of my talents, skills, or wisdom, but as the vehicle that has been blessed to use these in making the world a more beautiful place. I see my canvas as the world, my hand as the tool, and my heart as the inspiration that carries me higher. The artist is the Creator working through us in coloring the world with magnificent shades. As students of life, we must remind ourselves that the gifts we possess could have been given to anyone else. If we have been blessed with something special, we need to humbly embrace and cultivate it so it grows and inspires others. Humility is the soil for inspiration. It is the foundation of all good relationships between a teacher and a student. For a teacher, humility means being sincere, speaking from the heart, and being reachable. For the student, it is being respectful and open to receiving wisdom that can change their life. To learn well, a student may have to set aside all that they have learned until now in order to embrace a new teaching.

Ego has no place in either the transmission or the reception of wisdom. When criticism is given, we must let go of the self for a moment to listen and take in what is being said. Sometimes it is positive! As difficult as it is, we need to somehow embrace and apply appropriate changes to our life. We must be strong enough to not let our pride come in the way of criticism, nor must we be a doormat.

Before we choose to criticize another person, the sages advise to check our love for them and make sure it is perfect.[17] Moreover, the sages say that one is not in a position to criticize until one has reached that person's actual situation.[18]

Learning involves a bond of trust formed between a teacher and a student. Trust has a lot to do with transparency. The sages call this *tocho keboro*, meaning "your outer self is a reflection of your inner self." From the way a teacher offers lessons, the students will either embrace or ignore the teaching. Students can sense whether the teacher lives by, and believes in, the lessons being taught. To ignite the fire in the heart, it is always more powerful when the teacher is living proof that what they are saying is real. What greater love, joy, and satisfaction could there be than inspiring an individual with wisdom attained through your personal experiences in life! Each one of us has a story to tell, but what distinguishes a teacher is the one who sees the essence of their encounters and is able to transmit that as lessons to learn from.

A teacher needs to be sensitive to their students' individual abilities, and to speak to each of them according to their level of understanding. When words come from the heart, they enter into the hearts of students and anyone else we hope to affect.

Education is a never-ending process. It begins when we are children, and even after we have finished our formal education, we are still learning the lessons of life. However educated, intelligent, and experienced we may be, there is always much more that we can learn. How much do we really know about ourselves? Our body *and* our soul? Our environment, our family, and our friends? Our world? How deep is our awareness of life? At the core of these inquiries, we are really asking: How do I apply the wisdom of the answers to my questions and learn to live a better life?

Each one of us, at some point, becomes the teacher, the *Lamed*, or the student. We may take on these roles at different moments or simultaneously. Either way, we must remember to teach and learn with a warm heart, one that is open to both giving and receiving wisdom.

Breath: Energetic Shape and Intention

The kavanas *of the* Lamed *are feelings of the heart, such as love, compassion, passion, and understanding. It is igniting the fire in the heart expressed through your creativity and flow.*

The *Lamed* requires focus, harmony, and being grounded. The inhale of the *Lamed* is creating space in your heart to glow in your light and affect the energy surrounding you. It is the offering of the heart as a gift of light to the eternal light. It is being a channel that connects to the Earth as you grow higher into the energy above you. The exhale is the pressing down of your feet to the Earth as you plant rays of light into the ground. It is deeply rooting in order to shine higher. It is growing taller by lengthening, to connect the Earth to the light. It is the settling down of your heart as it spreads its wings wider.

The *Lamed* is the tallest Hebrew letter and has been compared by Kabalists to a tower reaching high up into the sky. In this way the *Lamed* is similar to the Upward Salute Pose, also known as the Mountain Pose, or *Tadasana*, with Arms Overhead. When coming into the Upward Salute of the *Lamed*, envision your heart opening wide and connecting to the infinite light. The *Lamed* is shaped by grounding the feet to the Earth and growing taller as you extend your arms above you and open your heart to heaven. Imagine your heart as the altar upon which the gifts of breath are offered to the Divine.

A heart opens us to experiencing feelings that are real and positive. As you inhale, lift your breath up from your feet into your legs, hips, spine, and shoulders. Stretch your arms toward heaven, exhale, and press your feet down while stretching your arms up and over your head. Inhale, and envision your breath blowing from the tips of your fingers into the infinite heart. As you exhale, let go of the breath into every part of your body. Imagine that you are taking oxygen from the infinite heart. When the heart warms the body, every thought, and each word and action, are affected.

A heart filled with understanding allows you to love others as yourself, to share in the pain and the joy of the people in your life. It is the kindness you show to all people regardless of their differences, and it is the compassion you have for those who are in need, whether spiritual or physical.

The inhale in the Forward Bend with Hands Interlocked is at the lifting of the heart, and the exhale is the slow folding forward.

The inhale of the Locust Pose is the lifting of your arms and legs and squeezing the energy into the midline.

To develop a warm heart, we must cultivate an openness to giving and sharing our heart with others. We also need to liberate ourselves from anger, stereotypes, negativity, and feelings that prevent us from coming closer to one another. The freer we are, the more peacefully will we perceive the people around us and throughout the world.

I would like to conclude this section with an ancient Jewish prayer, which is repeated every morning, that asks for blessings of a deeper rhythm of the heart. Each word begins with the letter *Lamed*. The words are: "Oh Master of the universe, open my heart (*lev*) to comprehend (*lehavin*), discern (*lehaskil*), hear (*lishemoa*), learn (*lilemod*), teach (*lelamed*), keep (*lishmor*), do (*laasot*), and establish (*lekayem*) your infinite goodness through my heart."

Body

Poses:

Upward Salute Pose

Forward Bend Pose with Hands Interlocked

Locust Pose

Upward Salute Pose

Create the kavana (*intention*):

Your body is a sacred space for your soul, and your heart is the altar for every gift of breath you offer. This is the main *Lamed* pose and is particularly important to the Salutations, because it warms up the body and uses all of its muscles. By lengthening your body from the feet to the tips of your fingers, you will create more space for your heart to shine.

Directions into the pose:

1. Come into Mountain Pose by bringing your feet together and your arms to the sides.

2. Root down by pressing evenly on the four corners of your feet.

3. Create an arch under your soles as you draw down through your heels.

4. Straighten your legs and squeeze your outer thighs together.

5. Scoop your tailbone slightly down and maintain your hips angled evenly toward the center line of your body.

6. Draw your belly in slightly.

7. Lengthen your spine and neck.

8. Broaden your collarbones and release your shoulder blades away from your head, leaning toward the back of your waist.

9. As you inhale, lift your arms out and overhead, your fingertips reaching toward heaven. Alternatively, lift one arm at a time into the sky as you open your heart upward.

10. Widen your arms as much as necessary if you feel tightness in your shoulders.

11. Relax the tops of your shoulders away from your ears.

12. Draw your lower front ribs in.

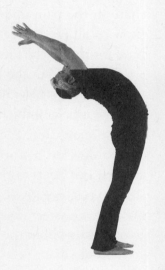

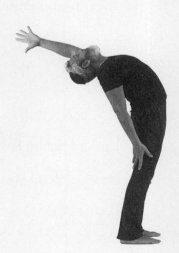

13. Keep your tailbone stretched toward the Earth.

14. As you connect to the heart of the *Lamed*, slope your head back gently, open your heart to heaven, and gaze upward.

15. Draw the center of your heart toward the universal heart.

16. Envision your heart moving your breath deeply throughout your body, energizing you with warmth and love.

17. On an inhale, lift through the sides of your waist.

18. On an exhale, soften your shoulders away from your ears.

19. When doing the *Lamed* as part of the Salutations, fold at the hips and move into a standing Forward Bend Pose—the letter *Yud*.

Health and benefits:

- Stretches the sides of the body, shoulders, armpits, and belly and lengthens the spine

- Relieves anxiety and fatigue, tones the thighs, and enhances digestion

- Opens the heart by creating space in the chest and lungs

- Makes space between each vertebrae, which sets up the spine for deeper movements

Forward Bend with Hands Interlocked

Create the kavana *(intention):*

Envision bowing down to your essence as you open your heart to receive. This pose releases the entire back of the body and allows the heart energy to expand.

Directions into the pose:

1. Begin in Mountain Pose.

2. Inhale, then exhale as you bring your hands behind you, and interlace them just below the sacrum.

3. Inhale, lift the heart high, and as you exhale slowly, fold forward. Remember that bending the knees is always a great option.

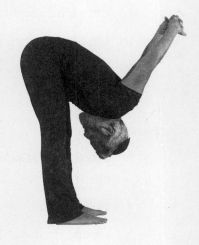

4. Work to soften the space between the shoulder blades as you continue to ground yourself through your feet, engaging the thighs and lengthening forward through the spine.

5. Stay for thirty seconds, continuing to maintain deep breathing into the points of tension.

6. To come out, push down through your heels and return to Mountain Pose.

7. Release your hands.

Health and benefits:

- Opens the shoulders
- Stretches the wrists
- Lengthens the back
- Relieves lower back pain
- Stretches the backs of the legs

Locust Pose

Create the kavana (*intention*):

Envision your heart lifting higher and opening from the Earth. This pose tones and strengthens the entire back of the body, creating more space for the heart to shine.

Directions into the pose:

1. Lie on your belly with your face down.

2. Place your palms on the ground next to your chest.

3. Inhale and softly press your hands on the Earth as you peel your heart up.

4. Lengthen your spine as you ground your hips to the Earth.

5. Draw your tailbone toward your heels.

6. Softly extend your arms forward and lift your feet.

7. Breathe into the pose and explore how high you can reach from your heart.

8. Inhale, and lift your arms and legs higher, squeezing the energy into the midline.

9. Move your shoulders away from the ears.

10. Keep your neck soft, as you gaze forward.

11. Keep your feet together and your arms at the level of your ears.

12. Exhale release, and bring your hands and feet to the Earth.

13. Repeat a few times.

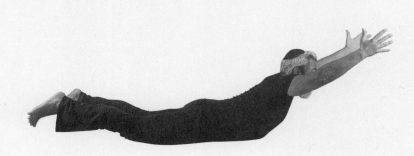

Health and benefits:

- Relieves back pain
- Increases spinal strength and flexibility
- Improves the function of the large and small intestines, liver, kidney, and spleen
- Stretches the spine, legs, and arms
- Opens the heart

CHAPTER 13

MEM: Sacred Space
Pose: The Camel

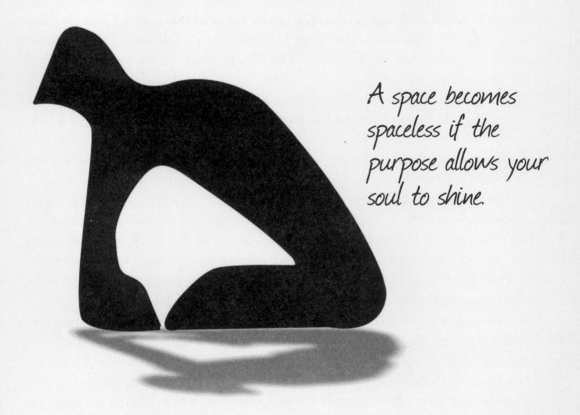

A space becomes spaceless if the purpose allows your soul to shine.

The *Mem* corresponds to the English letter M and has a numerical value of 40.

Soul

Mem: Mimarom Romo Vedar Bamerkava. "The sacred space of the universe dwells in your chariot (body)."

—Akivah

In the book of Genesis (chapter 28), the Bible tells the story of Jacob, the grandson of Abraham, who—after snatching the blessings of the first-born son from his brother, Esau—fled far away to an unknown land. On his way there, toward evening, he stopped on a mountain to rest. He gathered some stones, surrounded his head with them to create a safe place, and fell asleep. He dreamed of a ladder reaching heaven with angels ascending and descending. When he woke up, all the rocks had joined and become one under his head. He realized that this was a sacred place, lifted the stone from below his head, and said, "This space is awesome! It can only be the house of Elokim [a reference to the Creator], and the entrance to heaven."[19]

More than seven hundred years later, King Solomon built the temple on that mountain, and within it, created an inner sanctuary at the very same spot where Jacob had lain down and called it "the holy of holies." Inside this room was placed the sacred ark, on the very same spot where Jacob rested his head on the rock (which he later used as an altar) and dreamed of angels and a ladder.

The sages explained what was special about this sacred space: It was an open space that was dark, and in the middle of the room was the sacred ark. Inside it were the original stones upon which Moses engraved the Ten Commandments; the staff of Aaron, Moses's brother; and a vessel containing some remnants of the manna, the food from heaven that the people of Israel ate for forty years while traveling in the desert from Egypt to the promised land.[20]

The room of the holy of holies measured twenty cubits (an ancient measure of length, approximately equal to the length of a forearm, or about eighteen inches), while the ark at its center was two-and-a-half by one-and-a-half cubits. However, when one measured from the walls of the holy of holies to the ark, there were exactly ten cubits on each side. It was as though the ark occupied no space at all. Was this a miracle? Probably, yes.

For us however, whose lives are bound by the laws of nature, how can our own space become a non-space?

By creating a sacred space.

The Letter

Making a sacred space is the meaning of the thirteenth letter, *Mem*, which redefines what space is really about. Normally, a space is limited to its width, length, and depth. A space can become spaceless if we introduce another realm that is not limited to its physical size. The purpose we give and the intentions, *kavana*, grown in our space will cause it to be spaceless. Creating a sacred space is something we can easily do, and yet it has such a powerful effect on us.

It is the quality of the time spent by yourself in your own space that will determine its value in your life. Its worth will depend on what you do when you finally have that breathing space to find an openness for your mind to think more clearly, for your heart to feel better, and for your body to experience more deeply.

When we create such a space in our home, for example, no matter how big or small it is, we are inviting infinite space to embrace us. Such a place can be made by arranging an area in your home in a special way, such as a window view where the sky can be seen or an open room where clarity can be attained. It can also be as simple as setting up objects or meaningful things, such as an image of someone you admire, a lit candle, or an altar dedicated to helping you reconnect to your inner world.

In my home, we have two types of sacred space: One has a table and chair and is surrounded by the hundreds of books that fill my library. The other is an empty room with a few blocks, bolsters, cushions, and a yoga mat. Depending on the space I need to cultivate, I will choose one or the other. Usually it will be both daily, as my soul will be thirsting for some spiritual attention while my body will be wanting for more breath, stillness, and flow.

Because our soul is rooted in the eternal space, we have the ability to go beyond ourselves. We may be limited to our physical circumstances, but in our breath, we are spaceless. As long as the soul is in the body, we are breathing eternal space, and our ability to produce positive intentions, emotions, and actions is limitless.

The Kabalists explain that only a portion of your soul energy instills itself within the body, while its remaining energy, called *mazal* (translated as "fortune," another energy level of the letter *Mem*), hovers above you. *Mazal* acts as a reservoir of abundant energy unleashed each time we cultivate space for sacredness in our lives. When your soul shines in the moment of being in your sacred space, your mind opens to more wisdom, your heart embraces illuminated feelings, and your reactions are powerful and meaningful.

The letter *Mem* has two shapes, one that opens outward and another that folds inward. While the folded *Mem* symbolizes the inner world, the open *Mem* is the outer world. Both can be your sacred space if you make space for the soul to be present in the body.

In our sacred space, we can listen to the soft voice of the soul asking to be heard. When our inner voice talks, the *makom* ("eternal space") listens and guides us in our decisions and choices. When a space is made for the sacred, we create room for self-discovery. The letter *Mem* tells us that we can create sacred space in our *machshava* ("mind, thoughts, visions"), *midot* ("character, emotions, feelings"), and *ma'aseh* ("actions and reactions").

We need to make time to discover our inner self. Quantity can be important, but when it comes to finding space, it is not so much about quantity as quality. Such a place is found within our heart that whispers quietly, yearning to be heard. To give from our heart, the heart needs to be nourished. To nourish the heart, we need to make space for it to grow and express itself.

Space is that inner sanctuary where there is room for only yourself. In this private place, you are free to let go, detach, and release all life situations. You become you, an observer of the rhythm of life energy inside of you. Here you can truly think, laugh, cry, and just be you. In this space is you as you are in your light. Because our light never changes to something else, it is the only true space we can ever experience.

Breath: Energetic Shape and Intention

The kavanas of the Mem are feelings of spaciousness, gracefulness, stability, and openness of your heart. It is seeing your body as your personal temple of light.

There are two different shapes of the *Mem*: one that opens its center and one that is closed on all sides, known in Hebrew as *Mem Sofit*. While the open *Mem* symbolizes our openness to create sacred space, the closed *Mem* is the action of lengthening and drawing inward into this special space.

The open *Mem*, such as in the Camel Pose or Revolved Lunge, symbolizes a warm heart opening to the sky or to the side. In the Humble Warrior, the *Mem* opens downward into the heart center. The closed *Mem Sofit*, like in the Forward Bend Poses, is the act of bringing your heart closer to your body as you fold your upper body over your legs.

The Camel Pose is a heart-opening posture. It balances the heart and throat centers. Similar to a camel, the shape can take you on a journey into the depth of your heart. The inhale is the lifting and backward action of the sternum, while the exhale is pressing the toenails to the Earth. The inhale comes from the expansion of the chest and openness of your heart center, and the exhale is releasing your breath as you backbend into a cobra action from the pubic bone to the heart center, making more space to grow.

In the Revolved Lunge variation of Lunge Pose, the inhale is at the lengthening and twisting action of the spine as you turn your heart to the front leg. The exhale is the rooting down as your upper body settles into the twist, creating more space for your heart to open and your mind to be focused.

The Humble Warrior, also known as Devotional Warrior, is a hip- and heart-opening pose that reminds us to humbly look inward and value the space we cultivate in our life. In the Humble Warrior, the inhale is at the action of extending your spine from the hips to draw a line of energy to the top of the head. It is also at the opening of the heart as you lengthen your upper body forward. The exhale is folding forward as you go deeper into your sacred space with the heart leading the way.

The Forward Bend, also known as Standing Forward Fold, is a pose that relaxes the mind, while lengthening the backs of the legs, and creates space in the whole upper body. The inhale is the lengthening of the spine, while the exhale is bringing the navel inward. The inhale is also creating space in your heart, and the exhale is drawing the shoulder blades toward the hips.

The Seated Forward Bend is translated as "intense stretch of the west side." The inhale is at the lifting action of the upper body as the top of the head reaches for the toes. The exhale is at the rooting down of the hips and settling into the forward fold. With the palms pressed into the floor next to the hips, the inhale is at the lengthening forward of the spine from its base. The exhale is the torso moving forward, while the ribs come toward the knees and the chest toward the feet.

Body

Poses:

Camel Pose

Revolved Lunge Pose

Humble Warrior Pose

Forward Bend

Seated Forward Bend

Camel Pose

Create the kavana *(intention)*:

Make space in your heart by lengthening and opening as you elicit a feeling of love shining through your breath. This pose is a backbend that opens the whole front of the body, allowing the heart to shine and awaken emotions deep within.

Directions into the pose:

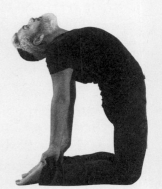

1. Come to a kneeling position on your knees directly above the hips with your knees hip-width apart. Push your shins firmly into the ground.

2. Place your hands on your lower back with your fingertips pointing toward the ground.

3. The power of back bending comes from the groundlessness of your legs. Scoop your tailbone under, inhale to expand your chest up toward the sky, and gently let your head fall back comfortably.

4. If there is more space, continue lifting your heart to the sky and bring your hands to your heels.

5. Press your feet to the ground as you push your hips forward.

6. Lengthen the tailbone down and release your head back, open your heart, and soften your neck.

7. Breathe deeply and freely through the chest.

Health and benefits:

- Makes space in the chest and lungs to breathe more energetically
- Improves posture, opens the spine, and strengthens the back muscles
- Energizes the body and helps reduce fatigue and anxiety
- Undoes the effects of sitting in a hunched position for a prolonged period
- Opens the hips and releases the muscles for sitting
- Releases the hip flexors, psoas, and rotator cuffs
- Stretches and opens the whole front body
- Opens the heart, which can lead to a major emotional release

Revolved Lunge Pose

Create the kavana (*intention*):

Make space by lengthening and opening your heart to the side and eliciting light deeply. The Revolved Lunge Pose is a twisted variation of Lunge Pose, which develops endurance and improves your balance.

Directions into the pose:

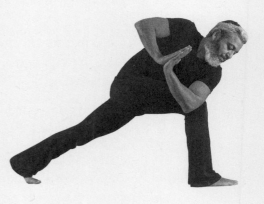

1. Come into the Lunge Pose with your right foot forward.

2. Inhale, bring your hands to your heart center, and envision touching your ability to love.

3. Exhale, extend your back leg, and draw the heel toward the Earth.

4. Inhale, lengthen your spine, and reach forward with the crown of your head.

5. Exhale, root down, and stabilize your body.

6. Inhale, and deeply gather air into your heart center.

7. Exhale, and twist toward your front leg, allowing your heart to lead the way.

8. Inhale, as you bring your hands together. Twist your torso so your left arm comes toward your right thigh.

9. Exhale, and press softly onto the side of your thigh to draw your torso closer to your leg.

10. Open your chest wide, gaze upward, and make space for your heart to rise.

11. Enjoy the space you have created. If you want to go further, extend your left fingertips to the Earth outside of your front leg and lift your right arm with fingers spread to heaven. Envision yourself as being the eternal space. Switch sides.

Health and benefits:

- Improves balance and concentration
- Stimulates the heart to awaken
- Develops endurance in the thighs
- Strengthens the quadriceps and gluteus muscles
- Stimulates the abdominal organs
- Stretches the psoas and hips
- Relieves sciatica pain

Humble Warrior Pose

Create the kavana (*intention*):

Bow forward into your depth as you make space for your heart to feel and explore its inner intentions. The Humble Warrior, or Devotional Warrior, is a pose that deeply opens the heart and hips and reminds us to surrender as we look inward and enjoy the moment of opening the heart.

Directions into the pose:

1. Come into Warrior I with the front leg bent and back leg extended.

2. Interlace your fingers behind you, and think of the magnificent depth you can reach. Inhale, and open your heart center, chest, and lungs.

3. Exhale, and gently bow forward with your heart open.

4. Inhale, and draw into deep feelings of your heart.

5. Exhale, and draw deeper as you bow forward.

6. To come out of the pose, press down on your feet as you gradually straighten your front leg and lift up. Switch sides.

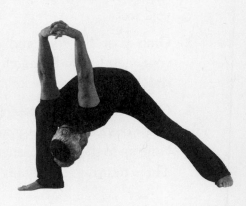

Health and benefits:

- Stretches the chest and lungs, shoulders and neck, belly, and groin

- Lengthens muscles in the shoulders, arms, and back

- Stretches and strengthens the thighs, ankles, and calves

Forward Bend

Create the kavana (*intention*):

Imagine that as you expand in the pose, you are releasing your inner light outward. The Forward Bend is a pose that brings harmony by lengthening your spine forward and down.

Directions into the pose:

1. Begin in Mountain Pose. Exhale, swan dive forward with a long spine, and extend forward from your hips.

2. Let your arms sweep down sideways with your fingers reaching the ground on either side of your feet.

3. Grab your big toes and exhale, lengthening your chest forward through your arms. Roll your shoulders away from your ears.

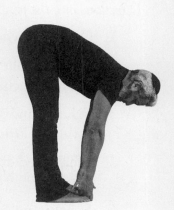

4. Continue to work opposing movements as you push your feet into the ground and lift your tailbone up to the ceiling, lengthening your heart forward through the arms. Then, return to Mountain Pose.

Health and benefits:

- Stretches the lower back and hamstrings

- Stimulates and rinses the organs in the belly, including the digestive system

- Brings a sense of harmony to the brain chemistry

Seated Forward Bend

Create the kavana *(intention):*

Think of the great space you can make in your body when drawing inward into the light that shines from your breath. The Seated Forward Bend stretches the entire body from head to toes, creating room for the life-force to flow to every part of your body.

Directions into the pose:

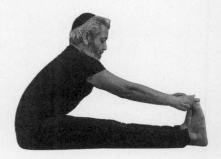

1. Start by sitting on the floor in Staff Pose with your legs extended.

2. Root down through your sitting bones and extend out through the center of the heels.

3. Bring your hands to your sides with fingers on the Earth.

4. Inhale, elongate your spine, and lift your heart.

5. Imagine that you are making room for your heart to expand to the crown of your head.

6. Drop your shoulders down and away from your ears.

7. Exhale and fold forward from the hips and over your legs while lengthening your arms toward the toes.

8. Inhale and grab your feet, toes, or legs or hold the ends of a strap placed around your feet.

9. Inhale, and softly raise and lengthen your spine with your heart open.

10. Exhale, release your body forward, and surrender to the pose.

11. To come out of the pose, exhale and lift your head and torso, curving the lower back.

Health and benefits:

- Massages the heart and reenergizes the spine
- Calms the mind and creates more space for meditation
- Stimulates the entire reproductive system
- Benefits the digestive system and rejuvenates the liver
- Relaxes the adrenal glands and tones the kidneys

CHAPTER 14

NUN: Creative Soul
Pose: Power Pose

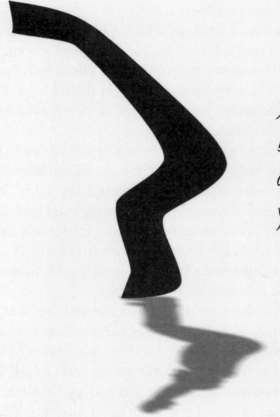

Your soul is your breath, your vitality, and the energy of your body.

The *Nun* corresponds to the English letter *N* and has a numerical value of 50.

Soul

Nun: Ner Hashem Nishmat Adam. "The candle of the Creator is your soul."

—Akivah

The sages tell a story of three men who approached the angel of fire and asked for his most precious gift—the radiant fire. The angel agreed, on condition that they would use it well and with purpose. The men went their way, and each had a different experience. The first man journeyed into a valley that was so dark that the people living there were frightened. Inspired to use the precious light, he gathered wood and began to make torches. Soon enough, the radiant light illuminated the valley, and people could see again.

The second man traveled to a town on a high mountain during a snowy winter night. It was dark and very cold, and people were freezing, some even to their last breath. The man immediately remembered the gift of light and built a fire, and the townsfolk began to warm up and heal from the cold.

The third man decided to preserve the fire from the wind, rain, and snow and kept it in a box close to his heart.

The moment came when they were facing the angel, who was eager to know what they did with the fire he had given them. The first and second men shared their stories of illuminating and warming people through the light. The angel blessed them that their light should always burn. When the third man spoke, he said that he had protected the fire from the world by keeping it safely in the box close to his heart. The angel felt bad as he told the man to open his box only to discover the fire had been extinguished a long time ago. He told the man that a flame can only survive is if it is being used to illuminate.

When the Creator contemplated making a physical world, our soul was the flame, *ner*, that shed light on the idea. For this reason, humans were created last so everything in creation would be finished and ready to be illuminated by them. Whether we are in a body or not, our soul has always been rooted into the eternal flame. The flame, however, is often in a box close to our heart and hidden from the Earth. When we reveal and begin to see from the light of the soul, we start to see the importance of each thing or person. In the same way that a candle can always share its light with another candle and not lose anything, so too we can share the light of our soul with others and never diminish our own light. On the contrary, the more light there is, the more there will be warmth, brightness, and positivity.

A physical flame is produced by placing oil into a vessel with a wick at its center. Both the oil and the wick are combustible, even though separately they could never produce light. For the soul's light to be revealed, a blending of human qualities is needed: a mind to meditate on wisdom, a heart to feel warmth, a mouth to speak truth, and a body to experience and share radiance. Without the light of your soul, none of these would be possible, and you could not shine in your body. The analogy of the candle tells us to illuminate in our presence, to shine in our heart, and to have clarity in our mind. These are the tools for kindling the light of our soul and bathing in its illumination. With every bit of effort we do to improve our health physically and spiritually, the flame within becomes brighter and a source of inspiration as we deal with the world around us.

Different from a physical light, the momentum of our soul light is not limited to a certain speed. Because the light of the soul has no material parts, it cannot be measured, shaped, sized, or weighed. Nor does our light have a beginning or an end, and so is now moving instantly toward the infinite light. For this reason, the light in your soul never ceases to shine. The light inside your soul can exist in space and still retain its infinite power. What alters the intensity of your light are the intentions you produce that lead to experiences.

Because we carry light, our duty on Earth is to share light. Like in the story about the three men, we cannot hold the light in our heart. If we do so, the light will be weakened and may even burn out. For a soul to be revived, it needs another soul to inspire it.

When the flame is extinguished, the fire never disappears. The fire always conceals itself inside the wick and the oil. To revive the fire, the oil and wick need to be united in a body, and only when they are together could it receive light from another light.

The Bible (Leviticus 6:1) says that the fire on the sacred altar burnt "at all times and was never extinguished." The Maggid of Mezeritch (Dov Baer, son of Abraham, who lived in 1700s), student of the Baal Shem Tov (Israel, son of Eliezer, who lived in the 1700s), once asked his students, "If the fire was burning all the time, then what does the verse add by saying it was also 'never extinguished'?" Because these words teach us that the if the fire is burning inside all the time, its light can overpower the "never" and "no" in all its forms of negativity, coldness, and darkness that separates us from being in the light.

Some of us are more in touch with our soul than others. The difference between someone who senses the light of their soul more than another is similar to controlling a light dimmer switch. It all depends on our intention, our *kavana*, which controls the dimmer switch of our soul. We can lift the switch and create more light, or we can lower the switch and dim the light. If our intention is to lower the light to see better, then the result will also be positive. But if it is lowered because of negative intentions, then it will be dark.

The Letter

The *Nun* tells us that the flame can shine into every moment of our lives. When we look inward to cultivate this fire, we need to reassure ourselves that the flame is being maintained by using it wisely.

Close your eyes for a moment. Breathe deeply. Ask yourself: Is the inside of the flame burning? Is it warm? Bright? A flame moves with thirst to reach upward, as if to detach itself from the wick and connect to something much greater, purer, and more spiritual. Still, it pulls back to its body, to the Earth, assuming its function to be a source of illumination within the physical realm.

The inner light of our soul is as natural to us as our body. When we open our heart and allow its oil of feelings to connect to the wick's mind, a flame will be ignited if our intention is to shine with light.

Breath: Energetic Shape and Intention

The kavana *of the* Nun *is to see your body as a candle and your soul as a flame yearning to surge upward and shine with all its light. It also represents breath, soul, light, inspiration, and a fiery heart.*

The *Nun* has two unique shapes. One, which bends at its legs, as in Power Pose, represents connecting to your soul. The other, known as *Nun Sofit*, is a lengthened vertical line representing the extension of your soul to the energy of the world. It requires strength and stability in your body, openness in your heart, lightness in your mind, and flow in your breath.

The main pose for the *Nun* is the Power Pose and is shaped by grounding the feet while bending the knees, extending the arms into the sky. The shape symbolizes a body rooted into the Earth, yet desiring to reach into higher realms. The inhale is at the expansion of the light of your heart as you lengthen your spine and reach your arms toward the sky. The exhale is the grounding of the feet as you settle into your sacred space connecting to the Earth, while maintaining a lengthened back with inner legs drawing inward, uniting into the midline of your body.

The *Nun* can also be assumed in the Power Pose variations, such as clasping the fingers behind you or above you. Bringing hands together is always a reminder that to shine, we need to be connected and become one.

Another posture the *Nun* assumes is in the Revolving Power Pose, a deep posture that grows from the Power Pose. In it, we use strength at the level of our roots to turn into a twist and allow our inner light to cleanse the world within by letting go of all unwanted and accumulated toxins. The inhale is at the lengthening of the spine while drawing the belly inward to create more space. The exhale is at the rooting of the feet and the deepening of the twist. Remember to always create space in your body before doing these two actions.

The *Nun Sofit* variation of the *Nun* consists of upside-down poses, such as the Headstand, where, when you finally are able to maintain this pose in the safest way, you can experience a great clarity and sharpness in your mind.

Each of these shapes symbolizes a different way for the fire of the soul to be channeled. When in the Power Pose and its variations, the soul gears itself to spread its wings and spread its light. When in the Headstand, the soul is lengthening to reach outward to heaven and to others as your breath becomes focused, light, and steady.

Body

Poses:

Power Pose

Revolving Power Pose

Headstand

Power Pose

Create the kavana (*intention*):

You are an elevated being who carries a soul connected to the Earth underneath you and to the sky above you. The Power Pose requires rootedness into the Earth while the upper body lengthens and makes space to receive the sky.

Directions into the pose:

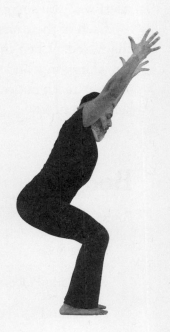

1. Come into Mountain Pose with your feet strongly rooted into the Earth.

2. Inhale, lengthen your spine, slightly bend your knees, and put your thumbs into the creases of your hips.

3. Exhale, and push your thumbs back deeply to create a direction for your hips to draw back, bending your knees deeper at the same time.

4. Keep your knees hip-width apart, hugging the energy of your inner thighs toward your midline.

5. On each inhale, lengthen your spine, and on each exhale, deepen your fold.

6. Inhale, and reach your arms up, parallel to each other, eventually in line with your ears.

7. Exhale, and lower your hips and bring the creases of your hips backward.

8. Drop your shoulders away from your ears and slide your shoulder blades down toward your hips.

9. Scoop your tailbone toward the Earth and slightly in, toward your pubic bone, to maintain some length in your lower back.

10. Imagine that a stream of light is passing between your inner thighs and hands, creating a constant flame rising high.

11. Press down into the four corners of your feet.

12. Ease your toes by lifting them up from time to time.

13. Stay in the pose for ten to twenty breaths.

14. To come out, push into your feet, lengthen your legs, inhale to stand with your arms up to the sky, and exhale as your move your hands to your heart, coming back to Mountain Pose.

Health and benefits:

- Strengthens the ankles, thighs, calves, and spine
- Stretches the shoulders and chest
- Stimulates the abdominal organs, diaphragm, and heart

Revolving Power Pose

Create the kavana *(intention):*

Envision creating more space in your body for the light within to expand. The Revolving Power Pose is a deep pose that roots you into the Earth and is a deep twist that cleanses your inner world, physically and spiritually.

Directions into the pose:

1. From the Power Pose, bring your feet and knees closer together.

2. On your next exhale, bring your hands together in prayer position to your heart.

3. Inhale, and visualize the great light inside of you and how bringing it out will make you feel.

4. Inhale, anchor your heels down, and lengthen your spine all the way to the crown of your head.

5. On an exhalation, bring your left elbow to the outside of your right thigh.

6. At this point, if you want, you can release your hands for a moment and actively draw your belly and organs up toward the sky with the help of your right hand. This will deepen your twist in a natural way.

7. To move deeper, open the arms, reaching your right fingers up toward the sky and your left fingers toward the ground. Stack the shoulders, one on top of the other. Continue to breathe deeply and fully to promote a wonderful twist of the entire spine.

8. To come out, bring your palms back to together at the center of your heart. Press down through your heels and inhale to come back up to the start position with hands above the head. Repeat on the other side.

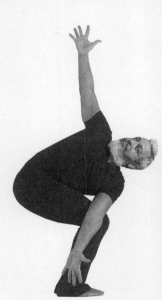

Health and benefits:

- Deeply twists the entire spine
- Strengthens the thighs and hamstrings
- Opens the heart and chest
- Cleanses and massages the internal organs

Headstand

Create the kavana (*intention*):

Envision light passing through you as you plant your roots into the sky and connect the crown of your head to the Earth, creating more space to shine brightly. The benefit of being upside down, such as in the Headstand, also known as the "king of poses," is that it is a great antigravity tool for all your inner organs, which brings more life, light, and oxygen into them.

Directions into the pose:

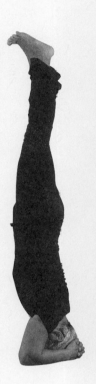

1. Start on your knees in the Child Pose. Lace your fingers together in front of you, and bring your forearms to the floor.

2. Place your elbows directly under your shoulders. One pinky finger should be in front of the other to create flat and steady outer hands.

3. Make sure the weight is evenly distributed between the wrists and the forearms, and that you are always pressing against the Earth to move your shoulders away.

4. Place the crown of your head on the floor between your hands and arms.

5. Lift your hips up, and start walking your feet toward your hands with your heels up until your hips are over your shoulders

6. Inhale, exhale, bend your knees, and squeeze them tight toward the chest.

7. Keep the knees bent as you squeeze the abdomen to lift your hips slowly and with a controlled movement toward the sky. Try to lift both feet together with bent knees.

8. Straighten your knees and bring your feet up toward the sky. Extend through the legs as you flex the feet and spiral the thighs in. Breathe deeply and work to hold for thirty seconds to a minute.

9. Slide your shoulder blades away from the Earth, creating a strong support in your upper body.

10. Keep your navel drawn in and lift your legs with a focused direction toward the sky, pressing the base of your toes up toward the ceiling, and squeezing your inner thighs toward one another, making sure your tailbone keeps lifting toward your heels.

11. To come out, lower your knees toward your chest and then lower your feet to the ground. Return to Child Pose and rest for thirty seconds to a minute, feeling the effects of this posture.

Health and benefits:

- Calms the brain and helps relieve stress
- Strengthens the arms, legs, and spine
- Strengthens the lungs
- Tones the abdominal organs
- Improves digestion
- Stimulates the entire body
- Awakens the nervous system

CHAPTER 15

SAMECH: Life Story

Pose: Dancer Pose

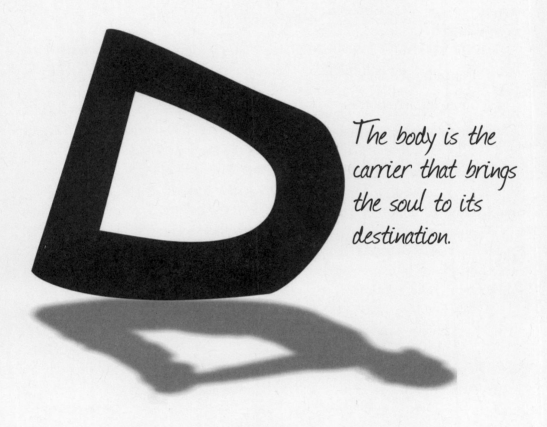

The body is the carrier that brings the soul to its destination.

The *Samech* corresponds to the English letter S and has a numerical value of 60.

Soul

Samech: Somech Hashem Lekol Hanofelim. "The universe holds you when you fall."

—Akivah

The Hassidim tell a story about Zusha, a great master who inspired many people to live a life filled with happiness. On the day of his passing, Zusha was surrounded by his disciples and suddenly began to cry. His students were surprised and said to him, "Master, didn't you teach us that we must be confident that in heaven, one's life will be viewed as those of Abraham, Isaac, and Jacob, the biblical role models?" "Indeed," he said, "but I am not crying because I am worried about being compared to the patriarchs. I am crying because I am concerned that in heaven, they will ask me, 'Were you the best that Zusha could have been?' And I don't know whether I was."

The sages explain that life begins as a thought imagined by the Creator. The thought is a powerful one that envisions you at your full potential. As the Creator breathed deeply into the shape of your body, the thought then became an intention to place a piece of eternal light in you. The light then became your soul planted into a fetus that embraced your existence inside your mother's body. For nine months, your mother was your universe as she carried your soul next to hers so she could nourish you physically and spiritually. As you were about to emerge, your soul was asked to make an oath to be the best that it can be! An angel then carved on top of your lips a medial cleft, signaling the universe's acceptance of your promise to live your full potential.

We are not born unprepared, as each soul is given tools to help fulfill its mission on Earth. These tools include intelligence, feelings, skills, and talent. The soul is also shown a blueprint of how it can be if it finds rhythm with the body. Each soul has a story that can only be told through the body that carries it. If we were to observe anyone from the moment they were born and consider all of their experiences, successes, and failures, we would have a perfect example of the soul's journey on Earth.

Will our soul story have meaning and consist of a unified purpose? Will our ideals and values link together? Will we see the light of wisdom streaming through the chapters of our life? Will we be a light that shines upon the world? This all depends on how much effort we make to embrace the life we are presented and cultivate the soil of our soul with the tools we were given. If we nourish only either the body or the soul, the other will soon grow hungry and expire. If we irrigate the Earth of our soul, then we will grow and reach for our potential. To live an inspiring story, the soul needs to deeply connect with the body and reveal its light through this sacred union of the physical and spiritual.

The Letter

The *Samech* tells us that the soul's journey on Earth is the basis of the story, *sipur*, that our life will tell. The soul always has a purpose to fulfill. Sometimes the soul comes to the world to complete a task; other times, to initiate something new. The soul moves into stages that will be affected by age, achievements, and health. Growth, challenges, and the wisdom we gain from our experiences will be the chapters that run through the pages of our story.

From the moment of birth through childhood, adolescence, and adult life, we all play our part on Earth by dealing with the challenges that our opportunity on Earth comes with. No matter how difficult life may be, never forget that you have the tools to deal with it. If, and when, you have succeeded in your role on Earth, give gratitude to the Creator for blessing you with a shining soul. Humility will attract your purpose and help preserve it once you have found it. Finding harmony between all that we do is the key to happiness. When a common thread is found between the disparate things we do and how they all fit into our life, one helping the other, then we can discover peace in our journey. If there is no harmony, then our challenges will feel difficult and painful, and make us disconnected. The secret of each challenge is the wisdom that will be gained by accepting the experience. We may even find the greatest joy and happiness of our lives.

You are the main character of your story and the one who will determine what kind of tale you will tell. Will your life attract love, sincerity, and truth? Will you care for yourself and for others? Will you rise to your challenges and grow from your trials? Will you make room for your soul to shine? Will you be the best you can be?

Awareness of your soul is about seeing that your life matters. The fact that we are alive means that we have a purpose and can make a difference on Earth. The contrast between one individual and another will depend on how much attention will be given to the soul's mission.

The *Samech* is our perception (*sabor*) of this energy that allows us to see how important we are. Spiritual perception is something that develops, similar to how we grow wiser in adulthood. Spiritual perception is having developed this sensitivity by cultivating awareness of our soul and how it creates the story of our life. If we cultivate sensitivity, we can see the subtle light that stems from our soul and inspires our mind to think, our heart to feel with more understanding, and our body to encounter more meaning. This sensitivity will influence our perception and reaction to the world, as well as help us evolve into the best version of ourselves.

It is from this spiritual sensitivity that you will begin to have awareness of your story. Your personal story is about living your potential and making your life matter. It is being present in your daily experiences and giving your finest when it comes to sharing your mind and heart. Your story of life should speak from the heart.

Knowing that you have a role on Earth is essential to living your best. As long as you are a body and soul, you have the opportunity to influence the flow of your story.

Breath: Energetic Shape and Intention

The kavanas *of the* Samech *are feelings of endless life-force passing through you, of sacred energy elicited from your heart to feel deeply, and of harmony in body and soul.*

The design of the *Samech* is a circle that represents infinity. The *Samech's* circular symbol, such as in the Dancer Pose and the Floor Bow Pose, teaches us about the soul's eternal life that never ceases to exist.

The Dancer Pose is a graceful heart-opening pose formed by a circle of infinite energy carved into your body through a line that follows your spine, toes, and fingers. The inhale is on the expansion of your heart and chest as your upper body connects to the energy surrounding it. The exhale is at the drawing into your navel and the lengthening of your tailbone backward. As well, the inhale is as you root your supporting leg and foot deeper into the Earth. The exhale is as you draw the energy from below to grow higher and go deeper into the pose.

The Table Pose with Extended Hand to Foot will give you the opportunity to stay longer in a powerful heart opener. While the main action is to focus on being balanced while lifting your leg, in contrast to the Dancer Pose, you need to be gentler on the supporting leg because it is the knee that presses down to the ground, not the foot. On your inhale, create space in your whole upper body, and on your exhale, gather the outer energy of your body toward the midline to keep an active inner connection and strong sense of balance. While you are stable in the pose, expand your heart with your inhale and connect to your center and core when you exhale, keeping your hips square and allowing the energy to flow in this beautiful circle of life.

The Floor Bow Pose is another variation of the *Samech*, where the infinite circle is formed with hands and feet connected. Your heart is the window that expresses your life-force, as your body is uplifted into the one light. This deep heart pose conveys your true self, without restraint, fear, or concealment. The Bow Pose roots itself at the level of the hips, while the rest of the body is elevated through lightness. It is also a natural pose for many children, and is considered fun, giving a sense of freedom and vulnerability. The inhale is as you elevate and create space in your upper body, ready to receive a deep and profound breath that fills your heart and lungs. This deep inhale also stretches itself from these organs with a sense of new oxygen and power entering you. The exhalation is at the pressing down of your hips as you root yourself to the energy of the Earth to rise higher as you initiate the next inhale.

Because the *Samech* helps us carve out deeper breath and space in our hips and heart, any of its variations is a great way to heal emotions and reach a unique moment in your practice of yoga.

Body

Poses:

Dancer Pose

Table Pose with Extended Hand to Foot

Floor Bow Pose

Dancer Pose

Create the kavana *(intention):*

Envision that through your heart, a circle of infinite light is carved into your body, connecting through your spine, toes, and fingers. The Dancer Pose, also known as Lord of the Dance Pose, is a beautiful, heart-opening pose that creates stability, focus, and rooting down of the lower body while lifting from the pelvic floor and inner core.

Directions into the pose:

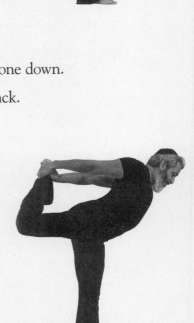

1. Start in Mountain Pose.

2. Take a moment to stabilize your stance physically and internally into a line of energy with both feet equally grounded.

3. Shift your body weight onto the left leg as you turn the left foot out to the side.

4. Inhale, bend your right knee, and grab the outside of your foot or ankle.

5. Inhale, and activate your thigh muscles of the supporting leg, lengthening and rooting down.

6. Lift your pubic bone, while drawing the tailbone down.

7. Envision making more space in your lower back.

8. When you feel stable and focused, inhale and allow your right foot to move away from the Earth and then away from your torso, creating a space of energy between your spine and leg.

9. Inhale, raise your left arm parallel to the ground, bend your elbow, fingers pointing up, and activate through your fingertips.

10. Set your gaze to one point ahead of you with softened but determined eyes.

11. Exhale, and allow your breath to flow into the front of your body, creating a magnificent space around your heart.

12. Keep your shoulders slightly back to enhance this flow.

13. Try to work between equal amounts of kicking into your right hand and reaching forward through your left arm and torso.

14. Hold for at a minimum of ten breaths, eventually reaching twenty to twenty-five, creating a deep focus on your foundation, your core, and your eyes.

15. From time to time, try to lift your right foot higher.

16. Eventually the pose can be done with both hands grasping the lifted foot.

17. To release the pose, bend the supporting leg slightly and gently release the back foot to the ground, taking a moment to stabilize your stance, before doing the other side.

Health and benefits:

- Stretches the shoulders and chest
- Stretches the thighs, groin, and abdomen
- Strengthens the legs, ankles, and spine
- Improves balance and patience

Table Pose with Extended Hand to Foot

Create the kavana (*intention*):

Envision that as you open your heart and lift your leg, you are drawing deeper into your essence.

Directions into the pose:

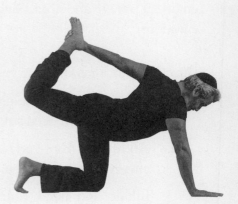

1. Start on your hands and knees, with your hands directly under your shoulders and your knees directly under your hips (in Table Top Pose).

2. Gaze at a point between your palms.

3. Draw your navel up to your spine, keeping your back neutral.

4. Extend your right leg backward, parallel to the floor.

5. With your abdominal muscles engaged, reach your left arm back to grab your ankle, and lift your leg toward the sky.

6. Hold for a few breaths, feeling the length of your whole body and connecting through your midline.

7. Bring your knee and arm down and do the pose on the other side.

Health and benefits:

- Strengthens the abdominals and lower back
- Brings flexibility to the spine, shoulders, and hips
- Stretches the torso and arms
- Improves focus, coordination, and physical equilibrium

Floor Bow Pose

Create the kavana *(intention):*

Imagine that a window is open through your heart for infinite light to shine out from your body, connecting through your toes and fingers, and through your spine and hips. This pose offers great energy to the body and heart as it releases emotions, stress, and anxiety, while remaining rooted in the hips, which carries emotions.

Directions into the pose:

1. Lie on your belly, taking a few breaths to get ready for a deep stretch.

2. Allow your front body to connect to the energy underneath you.

3. Inhale and bend your knees, keeping them hip-width apart.

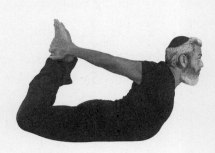

4. Reach back with both arms and grasp the outsides of your ankles.

5. Envision your body as the vessel for carrying infinite light.

6. On a deep inhale, lift your heels away from your buttocks and lift your thighs away from the floor. Your upper torso and head will follow the movement by being lifted away from the Earth.

7. Feel the lift of your heart reaching higher into infinite space.

8. Exhale, and draw your shoulder blades back toward each other to support your heart.

9. Keep your shoulders down and away from your ears and gaze forward.

10. Allow your head to move forward so the neck can relax.

11. Just as in the Dancer Pose, there is an equal balance between kicking back and extending forward. Be sure that the breath flows deeply and evenly throughout the pose.

12. Stay in the pose for at least ten to fifteen breaths, always enhancing the pose with each breath, and feeling a soft pulsation from within creating more space.

13. Lengthen your tailbone back to create space in your lower back.

14. Feel the breath in your collarbone, chest, and back.

15. Release on an exhale and lie still for a few breaths. The pose can be repeated once or even twice more.

Health and benefits:

- Stretches the chest and entire front of the body
- Stimulates the ankles, groin, and thighs
- Opens the throat, lungs, and heart
- Tones the back muscles
- Stimulates the internal organs of the belly

CHAPTER 16

AYIN: Inner Eye

Pose: Downward Dog
with Upright Leg

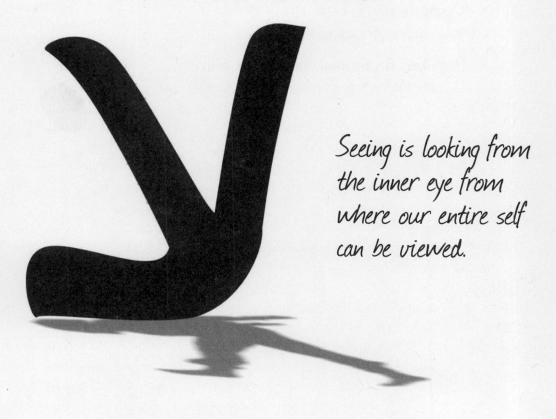

Seeing is looking from
the inner eye from
where our entire self
can be viewed.

The *Ayin* corresponds to the English letter O and sometimes A.
Ayin has a numerical value of 70.

Soul

Ayin: Ayin Lekol Ayin Vehi Orah Lekol Orah. "The inner eye of the eye is the light to all lights."

—*Akivah*

A story is told about a man who had survived poverty, tough times, and war, and had an inspiring life story to tell. He wanted to write about his remarkable journey on Earth, but his eyesight was very weak. He was nonetheless determined to do it, so for ten years with difficulty he wrote and rewrote the story of his life. Although his vision was slowly deteriorating to the point that he could hardly see, his desire kept him inspired. He was at the end of his book, and with great concentration gave every breath he had to the task. As he wrote the last few words, he suddenly began to feel faint and fell into a deep sleep. Upon waking, he could not see. His condition did not change, so his family took him to a special eye doctor. After many tests, the doctor concluded that the man had, in fact, been blind for years.

Our eyes can see in two directions. They face the outside world and allow us to capture all that surrounds us. They are also the windows to the hidden world of the soul.

When we see the world outside of us, we can view the external layers of life as well as its internal ones. Depending upon how deeply we see, we can see more than just the surface of things. Looking inward through the eyes is something different because it lets us see beyond our physical body to view the nature of the soul. Is it on fire? Is it bright? Is it warm? Is it passionate? When the soul is on fire, it influences our perception of what is outside of us. What allowed the man in the story to see for so long was that he was looking through the other side of his eyes, envisioning his soul. This vision ignited in him the desire to write his personal story. By going above his physical eyesight, he revealed a great inner vision that led him beyond what his eyes could see.

The Letter

The letter *Ayin*—Hebrew for "eye"—symbolizes our higher levels of consciousness, similar to the third eye or sixth sense, where our reflexes, intuition, and intentions are stimulated by bringing us to see beyond the layers of ordinary reality.

In Hinduism, the power of *Ayin* is known as *ajna*, or similarly *ayna* (because the letter *J* interchanges with the Y—as in Hebrew), a variant to *Ayin*, referring to the eyes of the soul.

In yoga, the third eye or sixth sense is located in the center of the forehead, slightly above and between the eyebrows. In Kabalah, the *Ayin* vision starts at the same place and reaches upward to the top of the forehead. Specifically, the *Ayin* creates a level called *da'at*, "knowledge," that allows vision to be internalized. At the level of *da'at*, what we see becomes part of our consciousness and affects everything we think, say, and do.

Normally, when seeing through our physical eyes, our challenges and trials can cause restrictions. From this perception grows the narrow impression that we are confined and alone in our troubles. The physical world appears much larger than our life can handle, and when we lose sight, we start to get comfortable living in this narrow state of being. Seeing only with our external eyes can cause pain and suffering. The eyes can mislead, as they make our situations appear negative and harmful. In reality, there is great wisdom to be found in all our situations.

Seeing from *ayna*, however, is looking to the inner direction of the eye where an expansive view of ourselves becomes possible. We see our challenges as opportunities to go deeper into ourselves and discover beneath the layers of difficulties a teaching that we must acquire. Not everything the eyes see is for our growth and emancipation. Not everything we see on the Internet or billboards, for example, is a positive influence. To embrace the positive wisdom hidden within our visions, we must activate our inner eye to bring us into the depth of our mind, body, and heart.

The eye of the soul offers more for us to see than the form and external appearances of things or people. We see energy—something not so obvious to the physical eye.

Everything has its inner and outer life, and could never survive if either were missing. Our contact with the world is therefore twofold. We are used to connecting with the exterior world, but we do not usually see the energy of the inner action resulting from our connections. Nonetheless, we also have the power to see from deep inside when we look through the lenses of compassion and love, for example. Then we are awakening the essence of what it means to be truly connected to one another.

The sages say that we were created with two eyes so that with the right eye, we can see energy that is positive, and with the left eye, we can filter and release energy that is negative. How does this work?

The *Ayin* inner eye is a composite of intelligence, thoughts, emotions, and feelings. It is the gathering together of all your qualities as you peel away their outer layers and reach deeper into them to arrive at their essence. Eyes perceive what is before them while the brain processes these impressions. The heart will then start to lift its antenna to see whether there are feelings that can be elicited. The body will then respond. While the right eye welcomes positive energy that will affect our thoughts, feelings, and actions, the left eye serves to filter, protect, and preserve energy that comes in and touches our soul.

Our life consists of many layers. Many of us live in several worlds of family, friends, work, pleasure, and much more. While some worlds are connected closely, others are further apart. The visual from our *Ayin* brings these worlds together, creating one vision where we can see the soul of what we perceive.

The mystic Shmuel Hakatan taught: "Within the eye, there exists a microcosm of the entire universe. The eyeball, whose shape is like the letter O, is the world, the white is the ocean, the iris is the Earth, and the pupil is the sanctuary you construct for the universe to dwell within you."[21]

The *Ayin* teaches that the whole world exists within you. The more you create within you a sacred space for awareness, the more you draw deeper into the soul, the stronger your contact with the world at the level of the soul will be. With your deeper perception that grows from the vision of the soul, you learn to experience a different kind of life that is not defined by external limitations.

The eyes are an opening for information to enter our mind and heart, where intentions are born. When an intention touches the soul, we open to connecting to the soul of our experiences. This becomes possible because everything that exists in the world also exists inside of each of us. When we search within, we enter the essence where we see at the foundation what needs strengthening and cultivating. When we nourish ourselves, we are also nourishing the world around us and affecting its energy.

Breath: Energetic Shape and Intention

The kavanas of the Ayin are feelings of rootedness and the opening of your third eye—ayna in Hebrew, which also means "clarity"—to see depth, soulfulness, love, compassion, and gratitude.

While the intention is to look inward beyond your layers as you practice the various poses below, each pose brings us to that vision in its own unique way.

When you plant your heart toward the Earth, as in the Downward Dog with Upright Leg, envision your extended leg deepening your awareness. The inhale is at the extension of the upper body while placing the hands and fingers on the

Earth, open like stars. The inhale is also at the extending of the leg to the sky, while lifting the heart to gather energy from the Earth and sky. The exhale is the rooting down into the Earth and the softening of the heart, belly, and hips as you lengthen your awareness into your depths. The exhale softens your heart and brings that inner release into your belly and hips, keeping that awareness of length. The exhale is the melting of the heart toward the ground as you plant rays of light drawn from your extended leg to shine through your fingers.

In Reclining Hand-to-Big-Toe Pose, you rest on the Earth, connecting to the energy underneath you as you lengthen your leg toward the sky and connect to the energy above you. The inhale is at the lengthening of your leg to the space above you. The inhale is also at the opening of your leg as you visualize seeing much more than from the eyes. The exhale is as you softly deepen the stretch by bringing your extended leg closer to you. The exhale is also at the rooting of the lower leg toward the Earth softly and bringing awareness to a lengthened spine.

The *Ayin* in Abdominal Scissors Leg Lifts is a reminder that our core is the center of our inner strength that brings awareness to all our poses. The inhale is at the opening of the heart and chest. The inhale is also at the lengthening of your leg as you stretch each leg toward the sky. The exhale is at the changing of the sides as you alternate extending your legs. The exhale is drawing deeper into your core.

Body

Poses:

Downward Dog with Upright Leg

Reclining Hand-to-Big-Toe Pose

Abdominal Scissors Leg Lifts

Downward Dog with Upright Leg

Create the kavana *(intention):*

As you plant your heart toward the Earth, imagine that you are extending a warm connection through your roots to the sky. Downward Dog with Upright Leg is considered a soft inversion that roots down to lengthen your torso and supporting leg to bring awareness to your extended leg reaching for the sky.

Directions into the pose:

1. Start in a Downward Dog.

2. Keep pushing through the palms of your hands into the ground as you lengthen, and on the inhale, lift your left foot up toward the sky, keeping your hips square.

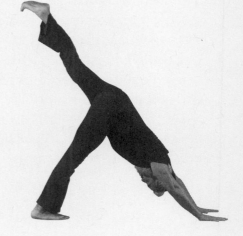

3. Keep an equal amount of weight in both arms and extend all the way to your raised foot. Breathe fully, and you can open the left hip on top of the right, creating more hip-openness.

4. Stay for at least five breaths, then bring your hips square again, and lower the foot back into Downward Dog.

5. After a few breaths in this neutral space, repeat on the other side.

Health and benefits:

*   Calms the brain, and relieves stress and mild depression

*   Energizes the entire body

*   Improves digestion

*   Relieves symptoms of menopause, headaches, insomnia, and fatigue

*   Stretches the abdominal wall and tones the buttocks and thighs

*   Brings relief to the lower back

*   Stretches the backs of the legs, particularly the hamstrings

Reclining Hand-to-Big-Toe Pose

Create the kavana (*intention*):

As you surrender into the Earth, imagine your body connecting to the life underneath you while your extended leg is free and connected to the energy above you. In this pose, you can connect to the Earth supporting you while resting on the floor to work your hamstrings and keep your back long.

Directions into the pose:

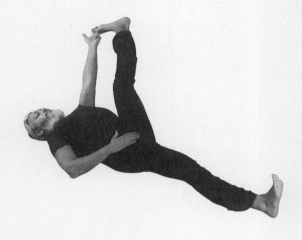

1. Lie on your back with both legs extended and pressed down toward the Earth, tailbone lengthening toward your heels. Make sure your head is comfortable; you can always add a blanket under your head.

2. Bring the left knee to your chest, hugging your thigh to your belly, making sure the right leg stays grounded.

3. Grab your big toe, inhale, and lengthen the leg up to the sky, pressing the foot toward the ceiling (you can also use a strap around the arch of your left foot, which will allow your shoulders to rest on the Earth, while creating length in your extended leg).

4. Exhale deeply into the backs of both legs. Work to extend and elongate the legs.

5. Stay for a good ten breaths, with every inhale creating more space and length.

6. On the exhale, smoothly and gently bring the leg closer to your torso, creating a wave of pulsations supported by your breath.

7. On an exhale, lower the leg and take a moment with both legs on the floor, feeling your breath. Then do the other side with the same awareness.

Health and benefits:

- Stretches the thighs, hips, hamstrings, and calves
- Strengthens the muscles around the knees
- Relieves lower back pain
- Improves digestion

Abdominal Scissors Legs Lifts

Create the kavana (*intention*):

Envision each opening in your body as an eye that allows you to see deeper. This pose works the core muscles and tones the abdomen.

Directions into the pose:

1. Lie on your back with your legs straight.

2. Bring your knees toward your torso and then extend your legs up, making a ninety-degree angle, pressing your sacrum down to the Earth.

3. Keep your palms flat on the ground with the thumbs underneath the buttocks, or for a greater challenge, place them behind your head.

4. On the exhale, firm your abdominal muscles by drawing the belly button into the spine.

5. Flex your feet, and by contracting your abdomen, begin to lower your right leg a few inches from the Earth. Then bring it back up on the exhale.

6. Repeat with the left leg and again with the right leg, creating a scissorlike movement.

7. Perform on each side for twenty counts.

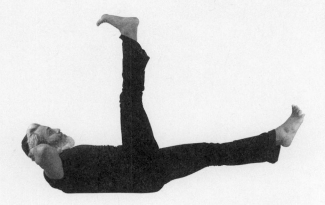

Health and benefits:

-   Tones and strengthens the deep abdominal muscles

CHAPTER 17

PEIH: Radiance

Pose: Camel with Hands on Lower Back

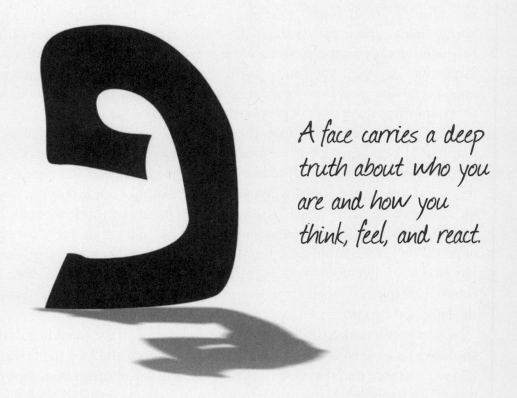

A face carries a deep truth about who you are and how you think, feel, and react.

The *Peih* corresponds to the English letter *P* and has a numerical value of 80.

Soul

Peih: Pitchon Peih Uma'aneh Lashon. "The inner face reveals itself through the flow of the tongue."

—Akivah

Many have asked me why I draw my teacher the Rebbe (Rabbi Menachem M. Schneerson) so often. It is true. If I were to count the drawings I have made of my teacher, it would probably be in the hundreds and represents about 60 percent of my art. Why? Drawing is one of my most sacred moments that I try to cultivate a few days every month. I tap into my creative soul where there is no limitation in time or space. If I am inspired, I can draw for hours, sometimes through the night or early in the morning when it is quiet at home. Space affects our inspiration. An open, quiet, and peaceful space is ideal. I draw in our living room on a special altar that I use for reading the Torah, prayer, and meditation. Most of my drawings are of faces of people who inspire me.

Michelangelo once said, "I saw the angel in the marble and carved until I set him free." I begin drawing by visualizing on the paper the face I wish to bring out. I feel my subject is already hidden on the white paper, and all I need to do is reveal it. Drawing the Rebbe is not just an expression of art; it is also a way for me to receive his light. When I shade his deep blue eyes, I think about his light entering my soul. His smile reminds me to be happy and joyous. Each soft stroke of pencil on his beautiful white beard brings me feelings of awe and reverence. His face is wisdom and opens me to embracing his teachings. A radiant face comes from spiritual moments that awaken happiness within us, as we bathe in the light of the source.

Did you ever notice the faces of a bride and groom on their wedding day? Or the look of a mother as she sets eyes on her newly born child for the first time? Did you ever gaze into the eyes of a person who had just returned from a spiritual retreat? Or someone who had just returned from spending time with their teacher of life? These faces all glow with joy and happiness. They are all shining through the face of their soul.

The Zohar says that a face tells us about the light of the soul, whether it is shining brightly, dimmed by shades of darkness, or glowing in another color. The word *peh* in Hebrew means "mouth," and implies that with the mouth, we can smile and radiate our *panim*, "face." A fake smile is noticeable. A real smile will be reflected on our face. Our *panim* will shine when it resembles our *pnimiut*, "the face of our soul." In the same way that the sun can shine light onto its subjects, the soul can radiate onto our face.

A face carries a deep truth about who you are and how you think, feel, and react to life. A face shows our challenges, sadness, and happiness. Because every person's face is special, no two faces are ever the same. Your face is unique because it belongs to you and no one else. It is true that a face is an inheritance from our parents and ancestors. Still, it is our soul that gives our genes a unique character, which affects how we look.

Rashi (Rabbi Shlomo Yitzchaki, the twelfth-century French exegete and mystic), in a famous biblical commentary on Exodus (2:6), relates that when Moses was found in the Nile by Bithiah, daughter of Pharaoh, what caught her attention was that he radiated with a brilliant light. Although he grew up as a prince and grandson of Pharaoh, he lived at a time of darkness and slavery, and so his light grew dimmer. It was not until Moses was eighty years old, when he discovered his mission on Earth, that the light he once had on his face as a child came back to him. The Bible says that when he returned from Mount Sinai with the Ten Commandments, his face radiated with a special countenance. Because his face shined so powerfully, it was impossible to look at him. Moses began to cover his face so he could be out in public. The only moment he would show his face was when he taught the secrets of creation to his students. At these moments, the students were face-to-face and open to bathe in the light of Moses's face.[22]

There is a certain radiance that exists in our teachers, mentors, and special people, that awakens in us the desire to bathe in their light. There is something very powerful about a picture of a revered teacher or saint that instills in our face the very same power. Very often it happens that we even begin to look like these special people who inspire us most, even to the point that our face and inner face change.

The sages say that the eyes of a person are the windows to their soul. The Rebbe had amazing eyes. When he looked into your eyes, it felt as though he had entered your soul. I remember how his face would change many times during gatherings. He would teach for hours before thousands of students, and depending on what topic he spoke about, his face was different. When he talked about worldly affairs, his face got serious. When he spoke the words of the Torah and ancestors, his face lit up. When he smiled, he could melt an entire room. During his talks, he would often stop speaking and begin singing a melody that was emotional or deep. On joyous occasions, he would often clap fast and lead us into a joyful song. He always made a point to look at you straight in the eyes during these gatherings and with a smile would say, "L'chaim," "to life."

The most auspicious moment came when he taught us the secrets. He would close his eyes, bow his head to his heart, and concentrate deeply. We stood while he sat during these moments, as we humbly received his teaching. These were sacred times, like with the students of Moses, when we basked in the light of our teacher's face.

When we find harmony within through joy and happiness, the face of the soul finds its reflection on our face. We start to see the world through the face of its soul, and relate to it with more depth. We hope to draw a smile that will come from the essence.

The Letter

One of the teachings of the letter *Peih* is that it can be pronounced as "poh," which is translated as "here" and teaches that we must be a presence and practice being in the now. It is not easy to live in the now. We may be here physically, but internally we could be wandering away. We often hide in the past or in a dream or somewhere in the future to avoid the present. We do so to avoid certain feelings or prevent certain memories from being awakened.

Being present will show on our face when we have awareness in our body, heart, and mind. To shine on our face, a special connection must be made with the source of light. We need to be awakened by finding joy and happiness within us. We are not always getting married or having kids. What we can do is create moments where we can meditate on all the things that make us smile. Remember the liberty we had as children when we shone with innocence and freedom. Over the years, the light became dimmer as we assumed our role on Earth. We must seek to revive the original light we once shone as a child and to awaken within ourselves the innocence and freedom we had in our youth. It is inside of us because we all expressed it at one point in time.

Breath: Energetic Shape and Intention

The kavanas of the Peih are feelings of confidence, an open heart, presence, and beauty. It is awareness of the Earth, sky, and life that embrace you.

The Camel with Hands on Lower Back is a pose that most resembles the *Peih*. The letter is about expression, and the pose reveals the heart's energy. The inhale is at the lengthening of your back with your upper body, reaching your heart up toward the sky. The exhale is at the grounding of your lower body as it carries the open heart that shines from within.

The Standing Backbend requires rootedness in your lower body and openness in your heart to the universe. The inhale is the connection you make to the

Earth as you press down through the four corners of your feet. It is also on the lengthening from the inside and the expansion of the heart as it rises to the energy above you. The exhale is with the melting through the lower body, releasing all the tensions and deepening to your core's center. It is in the feet where you are rooted and create space for your heart and face to shine.

The *Peih* in the Eagle Pose of balance and concentration allows you to go deeper into yourself as you cross both sides of the body connecting to your inner face. The inhale is at the rooting action through the supporting leg. It is also at the lifting of the leg that crosses over. The exhale is at the balancing and settling of the body, breathing into a space of peace, strength, and vision.

The *Peih* in the Cow Face Variation brings deep awareness of releasing energy toward the Earth, which creates an openness in your hips from sitting in an unusual crossed-leg pose. The inhale is the expansion of your breath, and it embraces your whole upper body. The exhale is at the grounding of yourself deeper into the Earth and the lengthening of your spine at the same time.

As mentioned earlier, the meaning of the *Peih* is "face" or "mouth," which symbolizes our inner face. The cow face image in the pose is formed by crossing the legs, which can look like lips, and the rest of the body becomes the face. The outer face is what you show to others, and the inner face is the private image that exists inside of you. The breath will enable you to stay longer in the pose, being enhanced with every breath you take. The trust that you create with this pose opens your heart to releasing your inner self, a beautiful reflection of sacredness.

Body

Poses:

Camel Pose with Hands on Lower Back

Standing Backbend

Eagle Pose

Cow Face Variation

Camel Pose with Hands on Lower Back

Create the kavana (*intention*):

Enjoy the opportunity in Camel Pose to allow the heart to lead the way to be open and shine out all its inner beauty. When this pose becomes more natural to do, it releases an energy of space, lightness, and openness, and creates a sensation of light that was concealed and needed to be released through your heart.

Directions into the pose:

1. Come to kneeling on your knees, feet and legs hip-width apart. Keep your hips over your knees, tailbone reaching down.

2. Place your hands on your lower back, fingertips pointing up. Keep your hips stable and over your knees. Push equally into your hands, elbows pressing toward one another.

3. Inhale, and start leaning back with your upper body, reaching your heart up toward the sky. Exhale, and ground your lower body before opening your heart more. Reach your shoulder blades toward one another to support the upper part of your torso. To feel less compression in your lower back, lift your heart.

4. Breathe into that open space, and after five to ten breaths, slowly release to sitting on your heels.

Health and benefits:

- Stretches the entire front of the body, ankles, thighs, abdomen, chest, and throat
- Stretches the hip flexors
- Strengthens the back
- Improves posture
- Stimulates the organs of the abdomen

Standing Backbend

Create the kavana (*intention*):

Visualize shining through your heart and your face, reflecting the infinite energy surrounding you and embracing your infinite energy within. The Standing Backbend is a beautiful mix of stability through your feet, rooting down, and the openness of your heart supported by a supple spine.

Directions into the pose:

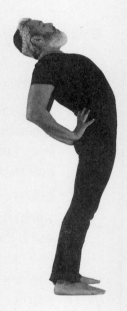

1. Begin in Mountain Pose. Separate your feet hip-width apart. Feel the steadiness of the pose.

2. Inhale, and reach your arms above your head. Exhale as you circle your arms down to the sides and place your hands for support on your lower back, with the fingertips facing up and your elbows pointing back and drawing energetically toward one another.

3. Root your legs down through your heels and tuck your tailbone under. Inhale deeply and begin to lift the center of your heart up toward the sky, keeping your shoulder blades well rooted to support your heart. While you exhale, keep your elbows pressing toward your midline.

4. On each inhale, let the space around your heart open, always trying to keep some length in your lower back to avoid too much compression. Stay for five deep breaths.

5. To come out, push down into your heels and inhale, returning to Mountain Pose.

Health and benefits:

- Strengthens and stretches the legs

- Relieves lower back pain

- Opens the chest and the heart, creating a more open passageway of breath

Eagle Pose

Create the kavana (*intention*):

Focus on your supporting leg being rooted as you find the balance in your body to be a center of connection. This is a balancing pose, which demands a lot of focus and groundedness. The pose might feel constricting, but try to see it as a deep inner connection to your center.

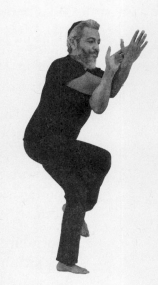

Directions into the pose:

1. Begin in Mountain Pose and bring the feet together, bending your knees slightly.

2. Bring more awareness to your left foot by lifting the toes and grounding through the ball and heel. Press the toes down and feel the solid foundation you created.

3. Lift your right leg and cross it over your left thigh. If you can, deepen this stretch by bringing the right toes around the back of your left calf and deepen your squat. It is important to use your focus and concentration to maintain your balance.

4. On your inhale, lift your arms to the level of your shoulders. Cross your right arm over your left at the level of your elbows.

5. Bend your elbows, and press your palms toward one another.

6. Keep a long torso, drawing your shoulder blades down and creating more space in the back of your heart.

7. Stay for five to ten breaths, allowing yourself to go slightly deeper into your squat while lifting your arms away from the Earth.

8. Come back to Mountain Pose and repeat on the other side.

Health and benefits:

• Improves balance

• Strengthens the inner thighs and ankles

Cow Face Variation

Create the kavana (*intention*):

Settle into the Earth as you root to the energy underneath you and connect it to the energy above you so that all is in harmony. When you do that, you will have more awareness of the groundedness of your sitting bones and more length in your spine. By creating that message in your spine, you create a clear space in your mind, and your face reflects that flow of energy, reaching up from the base of your spine to the crown of your head, bringing clarity, space, light, and peace.

Directions into the pose:

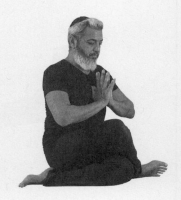

1. Start on your hands and knees, and place the left knee right behind the right, moving your feet away from one another. Lower to sit in the space between your feet, either on a block or on the floor.

2. Settle both sitting bones down toward the Earth. On your inhale, grow a little bit taller, and on your exhale, draw your navel in.

3. Bring your hands to prayer pose at your heart, then inhale, and extend your arms toward the sky, keeping your ribs and navel in.

4. On your next exhale, bring your hands back to your heart, inhale, lengthen your spine, and on the next exhale.

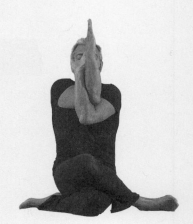

5. Stay for a few breaths, releasing energy down into the Earth. This will bring you deeply into yourself, giving you a chance to connect your inner light with the outer world where you will shine through the light of your face.

6. When you are ready, release the pose gently and repeat with the right knee behind the left.

Health and benefits:

- Stretches the ankles, hips, and thighs

CHAPTER 18

TSADIK: Divine Image

Pose: Goddess

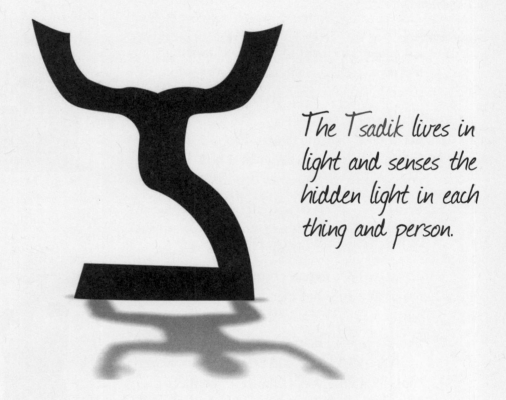

The Tsadik lives in light and senses the hidden light in each thing and person.

The *Tsadik* corresponds to the combined English letters *TS* and has a numerical value of 90.

Soul

Tsadik: Al Tikra Tsad Ela Tsedek Oseh Im Basar. "*Tsadik* is the goodness found in sacred man."

—Akivah

It was a cool fall day just after the High Holidays of Rosh Hashanah and Yom Kippur. I was a ten-year-old attending Yeshiva, an elementary school that taught the ancient Hebrew teachings, and we had been off for a couple of weeks to celebrate the Jewish New Year and the holidays that followed. On the first day back, everyone was feeling a bit lazy. The teacher told us to open the mystical work *Tanya* and to turn to chapter 1, which speaks about the *Tsadik* being "just." He asked me to read the first few lines. I remember this teacher, Rabbi Y, as a very sweet yet serious person. I began to read: "Prior to its descent on Earth, the soul makes a promise to be a *Tsadik*, a just person, and not a *rasha*, an immoral one. And even if the whole world regards you as a *Tsadik*, remain humble by seeing yourself as a *rasha*."[23] He then said to me, "Yehuda," my Hebrew name, "to take an oath to be a just person is one thing, but why also promise not to be a *rasha*? If a soul takes such an oath, it will think that by coming to Earth and embracing a body, it risks being immoral, and this will be cause for much unhappiness. How can a soul make such an oath and yet still serve its purpose on Earth with joy?"

That morning my teacher was singling me out more than anyone else in the class. This was not the first time, and I have always felt that this had to do with me being born into a nonorthodox family of North African descent, while the rest of my classmates were of Hassidic European descent. Strangely, being different has always worked to my benefit. I wanted to give an intelligent answer, and thought that perhaps it was to be found in the first part of the statement: "We make the soul promise to be a *Tsadik*," because he did not seem to be questioning that part of the teaching. For a moment I concentrated on the meaning of *Tsadik*, a just being, and then found the courage to start speaking: "To be a *Tsadik* is to be a righteous and good person, to help your fellow beings and to never hurt anyone. To be righteous is to see the right and positive in all situations, no matter how complicated they may be." I thought I was on a roll, but then he abruptly interrupted me and said, "How could a soul accept the possibility of being immoral?"

He paused, lifted his head up to the sky, and narrowed his eyes. He took a deep breath and, in a very joyful voice, as though he were singing, he began to explain:

A *Tsadik*'s soul comes from *atzilut*, the highest spiritual realm of excellence. He does not have a *yetzer hara*, a "negative inclination." He looks perpetually to heaven and always sees divine light in all beings. He is virtuous, and everything he does is with good intention. His desire is to reach out to every person and draw into their own light. He prays and meditates with passion and deep emotions. He has great awareness and always lives in the now. Because he is so connected to the universe, in him can be heard the Earth's heartbeat and the pulse of life. More importantly, because of his humility, divine light openly flows from within him.

He then stopped talking, looked at the entire class as though we knew the answer, and said in a serious voice, "Are you such a *Tsadik*? Can you be free of any negativity? Could you come so close to heaven and yet be connected to the Earth by caring for every person around you? Are you aware of your every thought, word, and action? Do you believe that such a person can exist? Can we see ourselves as nothing? Can any person be so excellent? So virtuous and elevated?" He then turned his head to the left, swung his hand in my direction, and pointed his finger at me. He said, "Are *you* such a *Tsadik*?"

The Letter

Everyone has a *Tsadik*, "just," potential within, the meaning of the letter *Tsadik*. We were born with a pure light, as the Creator chose to place his own perfect light within us. To be a *Tsadik* is to choose to cultivate this light of awareness. This is why the letter *Tsadik* is pronounced in this book as it is commonly known: "tsadik," with a *K*, the letter *Kuf*, because the authentic *Tsadik* dwells in sacredness. A *Tsadik* is known by the way they perceive their own life. Because their sacred being is evident, each thing they do is also from the perspective of sacredness. Every word uttered, each thought conceived, and everything done is with great consciousness and feeling. Nothing escapes them because everything is important, even the most insignificant things. The *Tsadik* person is a *tselem*, an image of divine light clothed in a body. Because the *Tsadik* lives in the light, they sense the light concealed in each thing and strive to reveal it. The *Tsadik* person shows us how to value all living creatures and to see how each and every thing contributes toward perfecting the light of existence.

A *Tsadik* personality is attained when we work on ourselves to elicit this type of energy, drawn from a higher source. The *Tsadik* never sees bad in any situation we normally would consider as such. Rather, the *Tsadik* sees it as a blessing so great that it is deeply hidden. Such a person blesses all that happens and sees it as an opportunity to cultivate more deeply the light within.

Pain is rooted in a higher source of positive energy concealed within us. Its purpose is to awaken us, to ask us to look deeper inside, and to reveal greater strength, trust, and positive thinking in order to overcome difficult challenges. To transform pain and fear into positive energy, they must be converted into *tsedek*, "equity"—the soil that makes up the heart of the *Tsadik*. *Tsedek* means practicing the qualities of the *Tsadik*, as we cultivate into the soil of our own heart the idea that one is all and all is one life-force flowing through each existence. To be a *Tsadik* is a process that can take many years and perhaps an entire lifetime. If we connect to individual people deemed as *Tsadiks*, we can be nourished from their energy as we learn to flow into the rhythm of life.

When this energy is awakened within you, it also begins to affect other individuals in your life. If your actions are positive, then they will create harmony and inspire others.

Because the realm of the *Tsadik* is where all is one with the source of light, the likelihood toward negativity is reduced. If we allow negativity in forms of anger, mistrust, doubt, and the like to enter us, the light of our *Tsadik* potential will begin to diminish. Good will not seem as good as we thought it was, and what was once real will now be questionable. Ego can also interrupt this virtuous way of living. A *Tsadik* personality can easily become proud and self-centered considering how spiritually advanced they may be.

Ego is living an illusion of yourself that is narrowed down to "I," "me," "my," "myself," and "mine." In truth, "I" is much more powerful when it transforms into "we" or "us." If we realize that the light in our "I" carries the same light that stems from the source of light, then it will become difficult to see our fellow beings as having a lesser light. What makes us different one from the other is in the expression of the light. Deep inside, we exist only because we are each rooted in the source of light.

The sages of Kabalah give us such beautiful insight into the stories behind the scenes of the Hebrew letters. The sages say that when the Creator was about to create the universe, each Hebrew letter approached the throne in heaven and said, "Use me to create." The letter *Tav* ("passion") came first, and the letter *Shin* ("peace") came second. When the letter *Tsadik* approached the Creator, it said, "Use me first to create, for I am the *Tsadik*, the righteous one, destined to be the shape that channels your presence into the world."

The Creator liked the idea very much, but he chose to begin creation with the letter *Beit*, to bless us with the gift of choice. *Beit* is the letter symbolizing the home and has a numerical value of 2, which also teaches us about being able to choose. Whatever our choices turn out to be, they will either increase or decrease the light within because we can choose. This is what distinguishes us from any other creature on Earth: the power to decide which way to go.

With this in mind, the Creator reasoned that being righteous can grow to an even greater level by first experiencing failure and weakness. The Creator responded to the letter *Tsadik*, "The *Beit* will build my home and provide choices, but you will illuminate it and bring all to the source of light. I will conceal your energy so that people will strive to seek you freely and of their own accord."

Breath: Energetic Shape and Intention

The kavanas *of the* Tsadik *are trust, sincerity, sacredness, honor, holy connection, inner depth, and openness.*

When twisting into the *Tsadik*, such as in the Spinal Twist, you are conveying your will to turn toward another direction that is more positive. When doing the Goddess Pose, you are outwardly opening to righteousness without fear of becoming egocentric, but confident that you are created in the divine image.

The inhale in the Goddess Pose is at the lifting action of the body when pressing down with our feet. The exhale is at the bending of the knees as we lower the hips toward the earth. The inhale is at the lengthening of the spine and the exhale at the rooting down of the tailbone.

The Spinal Twist is a beautiful pose of deep breath, giving a clear awareness of the profound twist in your core, making the space in your upper body more obvious. On your inhale, broaden your shoulders and collarbones and slide your shoulder blades down, making a safe support for your lungs and chest. Your inhale is all about the space you can create. When you exhale, bring your navel in deeply to accentuate the effects of your twist. Continue using this beautiful flow of inner life in your whole upper body, with your lower body being your foundation and root.

Body

Poses:

Goddess Pose and Side Stretch Variation

Spinal Twist

Goddess Pose and Side Stretch Variation

Create the kavana (*intention*):

Feel divine in your body as you reflect the space of the universe. This is a demanding pose on the legs, which requires a constant grounding of the lower body. The only way to stay and enjoy it is through your breath.

Directions into the pose:

1. From Mountain Pose, step your feet approximately three feet apart. Turn your toes about forty-five degrees out.

2. On an exhale, bend your knees until your thighs are parallel to the Earth and your knees are in line with your hips.

3. Make sure that your knees are over the center of your foot. Try to maintain a lift at the level of your pelvic floor.

4. Extend your arms out to the sides at the same level as your shoulders.

5. Inhale, bend your elbows ninety degrees, and lift your arms with the palms facing forward.

6. Spread your fingers apart like rays of light emanating from your body and bring your shoulders back.

7. Squeeze into your core as your lower ribs draw inward.

8. Extend your tailbone down to the ground and contemplate your connection to the Earth.

9. Stack your shoulders over your hips.

10. Open your heart, and remember you are a divine image!

11. With each exhalation, slightly draw your navel in and up.

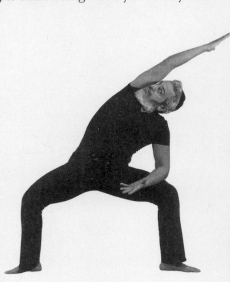

12. You can stay still, or exhale, and lower your left elbow onto your thigh.

13. Inhale, and extend your right arm toward the sky and over your head.

14. Exhale, and ground yourself from the hips to the Earth.

15. Relax your shoulders and breathe deeply into the space of your upper body.

16. To release, inhale, lengthen both arms to the sky, and on the exhale bring your hands to your heart.

17. Repeat the Goddess Pose and Side Stretch variation on the other side.

18. When you are done, come back to Mountain Pose.

Health and benefits:

- Stretches the thighs, calves, and groin
- Opens the hips
- Elongates the spine and relieves lower back pain
- Stretches the muscles between the ribs (the intercostal muscles)
- Extends the abdominal muscles and digestive organs

Spinal Twist

Create the kavana (*intention*):

Envision drawing deep into your core as you reveal your inner heart. The pose is about lengthening and twisting as you stay rooted upon the Earth.

Directions into the pose:

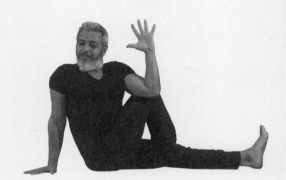

1. Begin seated with both legs extended straight out in front of you. Bend the right knee and slide your foot toward you.

2. Bring your right foot over your left leg, foot flat on the floor beside your thigh.

3. Keep grounded in your hips, and with a long spine, center your heart at the level of your right knee.

4. Inhale and lift your spine, and with your left hand on your right knee, twist to the right on your exhale.

5. Press your right hand down behind your right buttocks, and use it constantly to press into the Earth and keep the length in your spine.

6. If you have more space, bring your left upper arm to the outside of your right thigh.

7. Inhale as you lengthen up through the crown of your head, extending your spine, and exhale as you twist your spine to the right, drawing in your abdomen at the end of every exhale. Gaze where comfortable for your neck.

8. Perform this pose for five breaths, continuing to use your inhalation to lift through the chest and your exhalation to twist throughout the entire spine (lower, middle, and upper).

9. To release the pose, inhale, lengthen, and on the exhale release the twist.

10. Repeat on the other side.

Health and benefits:

- Improves digestion and increases appetite
- Stimulates the liver and kidneys
- Stretches the shoulders, hips, groin, and neck
- Relieves menstrual cramps and backache
- Relieves fatigue and sciatica
- Energizes the spine

CHAPTER 19

KUF: Offering

Pose: The Tree

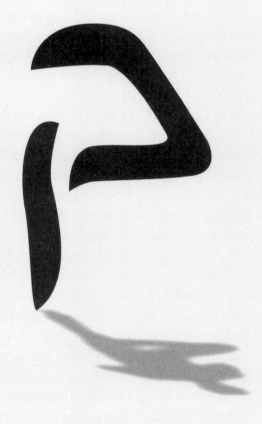

Holiness is being in tune with your soul's ability to shine.

The *Kuf* corresponds to the English letter *K* and has a numerical value of 100.

Soul

Kuf: Keroh Otan Bif'Neihem. "Speak from deep within."

—Akivah

When I was in grade four, my teacher, Rebi (Rabbi Schlomo Benarosch), would give us a lesson once a week in the Bible through drawing. Although he was blind in one eye, he was a great painter, always able to capture the moment. Each Friday for the first hour of the class, while we sang our prayers in Hebrew, he would draw on the blackboard with different colored chalks an episode from the Bible that we were to draw after prayers. As he gracefully drew an image of inspiration, he would also sing with us the words of the prayer according to melodies of Moroccan tradition. As we prayed together, we could not resist lifting our eyes from the prayer book to take peeks of the drawing being revealed on the blackboard.

At these moments, it was clear to us all that our teacher was not ordinary. Not only did he teach us how to open our heart in prayer and learn about the Creator and ancient times, but he also got us to work our imagination by bringing out creativity on paper. He wanted us to feel and envision what prayer and learning were all about. By the time we had finished praying, we had before us a masterpiece that we would now attempt to reproduce on our sketchpads. While we immersed ourselves in our creativity, art was being made through the vision he had instilled in our hearts. We drew, and he would go around the class offering us encouragement and tips for drawing techniques. Even my friends in the class who did not have much talent suddenly became artists. When we were done, he would then make us put our pencils down and tell us the stories behind these holy people he had drawn, and how each of them offered what was needed from their heart. He would point to the drawing on the board and act out the roles of his subjects. Once it was Noah and how he built the ark to save life from the flood. Another time it was Abraham as he welcomed three angels into his tent, and offered them a feast as they told him that at one hundred years old, he would have a son named Isaac. On a different occasion, it was Moses holding close to his heart the tablets with the Ten Commandments engraved on them that he offered as a gift to the people of Israel.

It was always difficult to erase the drawings he made. We did not want to let go of the image. Rebi's drawings were often so spectacular that all the teachers in the school would come and visit the class to view the masterpieces. Our classroom would become an art gallery for all to see and savor.

Rebi shared with us through our hearts, minds, eyes, mouths, ears, and souls what it meant to offer something to another person. He spoke passionately about holy people and how everything they did involved their whole being. He would remind us that a world without such individuals would be empty of meaning, generosity, compassion, and love. By noon, the drawing on the board was erased, but the image on our sketchpads remained a memory implanted deep in our heart.

The Letter

The letter *Kuf* is a beautiful letter that stands on one foot to teach us to be *kadosh*, "holy." Holiness is seeing the sacred in life. We are in the world but separated from the sacred because of attachment to materialism, honor, and fame. The holy person does not indulge in the pleasures associated with living as an ordinary human. Holiness is attained when we are so in tune with our soul that even as we are involved in the world, we continue to increase the light of the soul shining in our body, and rise in spirit, faith, and wisdom. The world becomes a platform for the holy person to blossom in its radiance and make others shine.

Holy is not synonymous with abstention from the world. We do not need to detach ourselves from the physical to be sacred. Rather, we need to be more aware of the holy energy that animates each person and thing. We come closer, *karov*, to the Creator by connecting to his creations. Because each one of us has a soul, we are naturally holy. For holiness to be shared, we must connect to others, knowing that they too are sacred beings carrying the eternal light. When we help another being from our heart, we increase the power of love. When we eat with more awareness, we rouse sacred energy found in the food and benefit from it so that we can survive. When we pray and meditate with feeling, we open our heart, mind, and body. Each time we give of our self to do things to bring happiness, preserve life, or spread goodness, we become a *kahal*, "a whole and complete body." The Creator sees us united as one such body and soul. If there is a pain in a toe, for example, the entire body will feel it. If the mind needs to get somewhere to share its thoughts, the feet will take it there. If the heart wants to show love to another person, the arms will stretch out and hug someone. When the soul needs to be ignited, it needs to be illuminated by another soul.

To be in the space of the *Kuf*, that is, of being holy and whole, we need to cultivate its most important character of *korban*, "offering." Offering and receiving the offering is what life is all about. Will we offer with awareness? A person who offers is viewed as generous, virtuous, noble, and kindhearted. A person who offers from their heart gives to others as they would want for themselves. We feel compassion for others who suffer because we know what it is to suffer and feel pain. Because we have felt or feel pain and yet approach it out of trust and faith, we find courage and inspiration to offer others.

The Earth offers us a platform to stand upon and build our homes and shelters. It also gives us soil so that we may cultivate produce in order to eat and live. The sun offers us light so that we can see, be warm, and have energy. The water lets us travel from one shore to another. It is also the vital energy for our plants to grow. The air we breathe gives us life to exist. It is also the one sure thing we all have in common, the need to breathe the air of the Creator. The elements were the first offerings and teach us that offering is a natural condition in all of us. The Creator is continuously animating the elements so that we may exist. When the wind blows, the sun shines, the ocean waves flow, and the Earth sprouts, they are thanking the Creator for offering them their life.

We can never learn how to care for ourselves if we do not care for the world. To be holy means seeing the light of the soul shining in all people. Wholeness comes when our offerings between each other cause us to grow physically, mentally, and emotionally.

To live in a holy way, we can never be without offering. To be whole, we need to offer and take back; otherwise, humankind would not function. We are dependent on each other. Whether from the baker, the mailman, or bus driver, we are constantly receiving offerings in order to function and return offerings so others can live. Most of us are always drawing in and out between our sense of offering and our resistance to offering due to the ego's feelings, which cause us to hold back or avoid seeing the generosity in the act. The unholy ego tells us not to get too close lest we become dependent. It sometimes goes further and makes us believe that if we give too much, there will not be enough for us to enjoy. Ego disassociates us from any sense of gratitude toward those who offer our daily needs. It plays tricks on those who offer by telling them, "Why give more if you can give less? What purpose is there in offering better quality, when you can give a lesser one? Is there a purpose in giving of yourself, when others can do for you?"

The more awareness you have of your feelings, the more you will have the awareness to feel for others. In your heart, you want others to succeed, and you do what you can to help them do so. By inspiring others to overcome their difficulties, you too begin to heal your own situation and come closer to being whole and holy. You also become more holy by seeing in your actions that you are offering from your soul to another soul. Such a flow of energy can affect everything, especially your efforts to reach into your inner self.

Concerning the daily offerings the priests of Israel were to bring, Leviticus (1:2) says, "A man who will bring an offering of himself to the Creator..." The sages asked, "What is the meaning of the words 'of himself' in this verse that speaks about bringing animal sacrifices?" They answered that the greatest offering one can make is not of his possessions, but of himself. Our body is a temple, with an altar made of a heart. On this altar, we can offer our entire self in every thought, word, and action, as an offering to the holy.

Offering is more than giving. It is acting from your heart without expectations. It is doing acts of kindness and generosity by reaching out to others and not wanting anything in return.

Noah saved humankind and was not awarded any special recognition. Abraham ran to offer his son Isaac as an offering to the Creator without expecting anything in return. Moses traveled forty years in the desert to bring the people of Israel to the promised land but never entered it.

Offering can be giving of our heart the pure essence of love, compassion, and understanding and not expecting to gain anything in return. It takes from our time, energy, and money, but we still offer because we care and want to make a difference in someone's life. We feel their difficulty and deal with it as though it were our own, personally. Offering tells us that humans need to be together and not apart. Apart we are nothing, not even our true selves. By being together and sharing with each other, we become one.

Life is sacred, and when we begin to see it this way, we invite the universe to open its heart to us. When we volunteer for causes, give time to friends, or help someone who needs a hand, we are connecting to the universe and completing the circle of life. There is so much we can give. We need to simply start seeing and feeling when we offer. Remember that every good thought, positive word, and generous action can make a difference and be an offering.

Breath: Energetic Shape and Intention

The kavanas of the Kuf are feelings of gratitude; closeness to others; connection to the Earth, sky, and energy around us; holiness; sacredness; and balance.

The Kuf in the Tree Pose represents our desire to grow like a tree toward heaven. To assume the *Kuf*, the supporting leg must be rooted to the ground with the hands placed either on the heart or extended upward or outward. Everything begins from the Earth, and when we plant our foundation into the ground, we are embracing its energy, from which all things grow.

When the hands are on the heart, it means that we take into our heart the feeling of being elevated. When the arms are extended, we are reaching for sacredness, and when out to the sides, we are hugging the universe and drawing its light into our heart. Whichever way you express yourself in the *Kuf*, the idea is to offer from deep inside your heart. The breath will carry this energy to bring life to the rest of the body.

When you inhale, you dig deeper into the life of the Earth and lift it up all the way to the crown of your head. When you exhale, it's always about rooting down into your roots and rooting into your inner core. When the arms are extended, allow every inhale to start deep in your core and travel all the way to your fingertips. Draw your ribs and your navel in on the exhale, and root your tailbone down.

The Head-to-Knee Pose allows you to connect with the Earth in a deep way, which releases tensions and restrictions. This deep forward bend allows you to go deep into your inner and private self, where only you can travel without any judgment, discovering your inner gems. The inhale will be the expansion of your whole body, while every exhalation brings you closer to yourself.

Softly inhaling and connecting to the space of your belly and exhaling and drawing your navel in is all done with softness and awareness. You can also focus a little bit more on every exhalation to deepen your stretch, and really allow your breath to travel deep into your hips, melting all the tensions away.

Body

Poses:

Tree Pose and Extended Tree Pose

Head-to-Knee Pose

Tree Pose and Extended Tree Pose

Create the kavana *(intention):*

Envision rising into the higher realms as you ground yourself deeper to the Earth and cultivate your potential. The Tree Pose is all about rootedness—gathering the energy of your roots into the Earth and filling it up throughout your body. In the extended variation, you can lengthen your breath with your arms extended like branches, revealing the beautiful rhythm of life in you.

Directions into the pose:

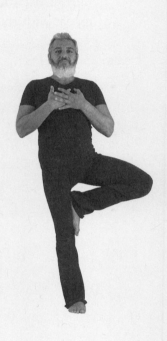

1. Begin in Mountain Pose.

2. Shift your weight slightly onto the right foot, and bend your left knee. Clasp your left ankle with your right hand and bring the sole of your foot to your inner right thigh.

3. Press the sole into your inner thigh and the inner thigh against the sole of your foot to create a stable balance and connection toward your midline.

4. Bring your hands to the center of your heart—either with the palms together in prayer position or palms flat against your chest, stacked one on top of the other. Roll your shoulders down the back and place them into their sockets.

5. Lengthen the crown of your head toward the sky.

6. Keep stable through the standing leg by rooting your foot into the ground and lifting the thigh muscle up and back. Press the bent knee back to keep the hip open.

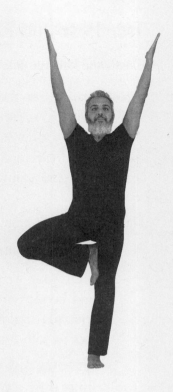

7. To come into the Extended Tree Pose, inhale and reach your arms toward the sky, always keeping space between your ears and your shoulders and drawing your shoulder blades down.

8. Keep your ribs and navel drawn in, while extending your whole upper body and deeply rooting from your tailbone down into the Earth.

9. After a few deep breaths, lower your palms to your heart, and release in Mountain Pose. Then repeat with the other leg.

Health and benefits:

- Promotes awareness of general posture and improves a sense of balance

- Lengthens the spine, and tones the legs

- Tone the sides of the upper body and opens the shoulders

- Calms the brain

Head-to-Knee Pose

Create the kavana (*intention*):

Visualize going deeper into your inner self as you awaken the sacredness within and beyond. This pose can be a blissful, restorative pose, where the breath can flow freely throughout your body.

Directions into the pose:

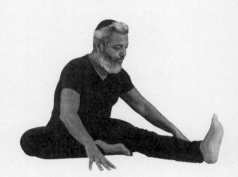

1. Begin with your legs straight out in front of you in Staff Pose, with the backs of your legs pressing into the floor.

2. Place your hands on the floor beside your hips, lifting your upper body, lower belly, and sides of your waist.

3. Bend your right knee and place your right foot against your left inner thigh, allowing your right knee to open away from your left thigh.

4. Lift your right arm up on an inhale, and twist to the left. Reach your arm to the outside of your left leg. Your hand will reach either the outside of your thigh or lower leg or maybe your ankle, but always allow your heart to be open.

5. When you inhale, lengthen your spine, and on your exhale, twist a little bit deeper.

6. Now you can slide your left hand toward the outside of your left foot and, keeping your heart in the direction of your left knee, release your right hand to place it on the inside of your left foot.

7. Inhale and lift your upper body away from your leg.

8. Exhale, melt, and dive a little bit deeper.

9. Stay for a few breaths, allowing a deep release, and then softly slide your hands back.

10. Come up vertebra by vertebra all the way to a long spine.

11. Breathe in Staff Pose and change sides.

Health and benefits:

- Stretches the hamstrings and the front of the legs
- Declutters the brain
- Stretches and stimulates the skin of the sides of the torso
- Can help lower blood pressure

CHAPTER 20

REISH: Pleasure

Pose: Standing Side Bend

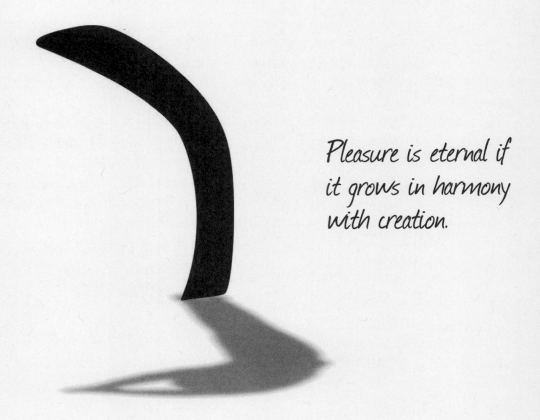

Pleasure is eternal if it grows in harmony with creation.

The *Reish* corresponds to the English letter *R* and has a numerical value of 200.

Soul

Reish: Reyach Nicho'ach L'Hashem. "A pleasurable fragrance is a sacred offering."

—Akivah

Adam, the first man on Earth, was part human and part spirit. The book of Genesis says that Adam was formed on the sixth day of creation so he would come into a world ready to be enjoyed and have everything he needed to fulfill his mission on Earth. He was formed out of the soil of the Earth, which came from every corner of the planet, so that man would symbolically represent all future humans wherever they would be. The Earth is said to have been mixed with water flowing from the great oceans and made into a clay. The clay was then molded into the shape of a human body. The moment came for man to be alive. The Creator drew divine breath from his innermost essence and "breathed it into Adam's nostrils" to "become a living soul" (Genesis 2:7).

We are born with an inhalation, and we die with an exhalation. The inhalation is the glowing of the light of your soul; the exhalation is the light of your soul detaching from your body as it joins its source of light. During our lifetime, we increase and dim the light by taking in the divine breath. When we exhale, we share this universal breath with the world by shining the light of the soul through our words and actions.

The soul is a piece of the Divine that came from the Creator's innermost thoughts and feelings as a form of consciousness. Humankind was given a soul and a body in order to receive light and spread light into the world. This energetic light, say the Kabalists, is given to each of us individually as we are born into this world.

Because Adam received *ruach*, "spirit," the meaning of the letter *Reish*, directly from the mouth of the Creator, he was given a unique soul. The animals, birds, and creatures, on the other hand, were not given *ruach* in such a direct way. Instead, they were formed as categories of souls based on their species. Thus, the birds were created from a *ruach* that allowed them to fly and sing, the cows were blessed with the ability to nourish by producing milk in abundance, the horses were given a soul to gallop and be joyful, and so on. Each category has its advantages and intelligence. What all categories have in common is their instinctual behavior. Adam, however, possessed a unique soul that allowed him to evolve physically and spiritually, and to reach higher levels of consciousness. For this reason, Adam was the most perfect creation that came into the world.

Physically he was beautiful, and mentally he was the most intelligent. He had the ability to sense the divine breath in each creature and see it as part of his own. Because man was made to be rooted deeply into the essence, he was auto-matically connected to each level of life on Earth.

Still, man was lonely. The Creator realized that Adam needed a companion to complete him (Genesis 2:18). Because man's awareness was superior to all creatures, in that he could perceive the divine essence in all forms of life, none of the other creatures were suitable to be his partner on Earth in fulfilling his mission. There needed to be an equal to man, both in spiritual and physical powers.

The Creator then put Adam to sleep and began to breathe his *ruach* into him. On a deep inhale, he took one of Adam's ribs out of his body, and on an exhale, he formed it into the shape of a woman and named her Chava, or Eve, meaning "living being."[24] Eve's body and soul possessed the energy magnitude of Adam but were formed differently, giving her marvelous wisdom that man did not have and the ability to bear children.[25]

Although Adam was the most perfect creation, Eve was made physically superior, and spiritually was given a higher *bina*, a level of understanding that only a woman has. To make her desirous to Adam, the Creator braided Eve's hair and presented her adorned with twenty-four ornaments.[26]

When Adam woke from the deep sleep, he saw Eve and immediately recog-nized in her his other half. He sensed that she possessed the indwelling of the one necessary to fulfill mankind's mission on Earth.

Adam and Eve lived in the most precious area on Earth, known as the Garden of Eden. The air was perfect. The garden was filled with incredible fra-grances, *reyach*, another meaning of the *Reish*, which had grown from the great *ruach* that had caused everything to grow, exist, and be. The *reyach*, fragrances of the garden, were derived from the pleasantness of the Earth, flowers, and trees. Spiritually, Adam's soul was eternal, and when he breathed in Eden, he could smell the fragrances that came from the higher worlds.

Each breath he took brought him to a deeper awareness of the one con-sciousness in all of life. Breathing in the garden made Adam and Eve more enlightened, as the oxygen came directly from the essence of the Creator. They were awakened through the scent and beauty surrounding them.

It was called Eden, meaning pleasure, because it was to be a place where Adam and Eve could have the utmost divine pleasure. Eden was a magnificent garden that had many trees bearing luscious fruits. The landscape was covered with green grass and fruits blossoming directly from the Earth. Four rivers flowed into Eden, namely, Pishon, Gihon, Tigris, and Euphrates, which naturally irri-gated the soil that caused everything to grow.

Awareness was so powerful in Eden that one could hear and feel the Creator moving the Earth and breathing the winds. When the sun shined brilliantly, all the creatures felt the Creator's warm heart.

Adam and Eve were pure and innocent, and walked around the garden naked. There was no such thing as bad thoughts or wrongdoing. Instead, Adam and Eve continued to evolve in their *ruach*, "essence," as they breathed the *reyach*, the smell of the higher realms, and took pleasure from it.

The Bible says that Adam and Eve were given two requests by the Creator, to "work and guard." The sages explain that "work" in Eden meant to serve the Creator by specifically savoring all the fruits in the garden. This did not mean plowing or irrigating the Earth. Rather, the garden was growing and blossoming on its own.

Why eat the fruits of the trees? Adam and Eve were to remind themselves that man is like a tree having roots, a body, branches, and the ability to bear fruits.[27] If humankind is rooted into the soil of *ruach*, the essence of life, then they will grow and be in harmony with the universe. If humankind is flowing with Creation, then the fruits humans will enjoy will also be pleasurable for the universe. If they are not rooted and lack consciousness of the One, then the changes of the seasons and challenges of life will destabilize them and move them into other directions that are not aligned with the will of the universe. Without awareness of the one essence, pleasure will no longer be as enjoyable.

To "guard" was the other request the Creator made of Adam and Eve: "Do not eat from the fruits of the tree of knowledge of good and bad" (Genesis 2:17), for this was not in his light. The Creator made a thing outside of his light so humankind could make a choice to be in harmony with him or not.[28]

Adam and Eve began to feel limited in their work. The fruits of the garden were not as attractive or tasty anymore. They wanted to try something different, and thought that by tasting from the fruit of the tree of knowledge, they could attain higher levels in their work of cultivating holiness.[29]

Rather than enjoying all the fruits of the Earth, Adam and Eve chose to eat fruits that were not permissible. A snake in the garden had convinced them to eat from the tree, making them believe that they would be spiritually elevated.

The Letter

The *Reish* teaches us that a world of pleasure, another meaning of *Reish*, cannot be without limitations. Boundaries are not always restrictions to our enjoyments, but limitations to some if they are done to preserve freedom. A free world needs boundaries so that people can live, enjoy, and be free, provided they are done with a purpose that honors life.

Our countries, cities, and societies set laws and regulations to preserve the freedoms that come from our membership and ensure that we have the full benefit of our pleasures. If there were no boundaries, then anyone's expression of pleasure could become an infringement on another person's pleasure and freedom. Pleasure does not mean that we can take or do as much as we want. It becomes infinite as long as we are enjoying within our own boundaries. Adam and Eve erred in that they forgot that pleasure is sacred and that Earth is a vessel to experiencing *reyach nichoach*, a "holy pleasure."

Awesome souls like those of the first man and woman must also make choices between good and bad. Our leaders, guides, and masters, who have the power to influence thousands or perhaps millions of lives, must also confront the boundaries of the pleasure that comes from good and bad. Adam and Eve taught us to see our pleasures as potentially sacred. Their eating of the forbidden fruit reminds us of our humanity and weaknesses. If this were not the case, we would not have the ability to choose. When we decide to be in alignment with the universe, our pleasures become the pleasures of the higher realms. And when the universe has pleasure, then all we do becomes a blessing in our lives.

Breath: Energetic Shape and Intention

The kavanas of the Reish are feelings of divinity, pleasure, lightness, freedom, gracefulness, rooting, and openness of your inner life. It is awareness of the energy surrounding you, below you, and above you.

The inspiration we get from the letter *Reish* is a great one, which applies not only to shaping the body into its postures but also to all of our yoga poses. Each letter we do has wisdom, beauty, and healing, and practicing yoga with intention allows for the divine essence to manifest itself in our yoga practice.

The shape of the *Reish* is like that of a wind blowing from side to side. With your feet rooted deeply into the Earth, the spine long, and the arms extended upward, your upper body is softened to open to the left and then to the right as a symbol of exploring your inner inspiration in all directions.

Because standing side bends are not part of our daily activities, the Standing Side Bend Pose is a perfect one to stretch out your body using your breath, as a way of illuminating the sides and the back of your body. The inhale is the lengthening of the spine and of the arms as you move your inner light toward the sky and from side to side. The exhale is at the foundations as you root deeply into your sacred space underneath you, while maintaining a lengthened spine moving from side to side.

In the Side Plank Variation, the inhale is the lifting action as you draw a horizontal line from the toes to the top of the head. It is also at the opening of the heart as the supporting hand presses down and the extended arm stretches overhead. On the exhale, maintain the lifting action, as you root down from the outer edge of the lower foot and press the upper foot down. The exhale is also internalizing through your core the energy within, which allows you to shine from your essence throughout the body.

The Wild Thing requires both strength of arms and softness of heart. Its power is that it combines both of these opposites simultaneously, making this pose unique. The inhale is at the lifting action of the body as the arms reach over the head toward the Earth. It is also at the opening of the heart and softening of the entire body as you expand in all directions. The exhale is at the grounding and strengthening of your foundation to the Earth as you blossom.

The power of breath is that it unites us to both our body and our soul as we bring more awareness to the action of our breath. The mystics call this movement *ratsu veshuv*, meaning expansion and contraction of the breath, body, and spirit.

Body

Poses:

Standing Side Bend Pose

Side Plank Variation

Wild Thing

Standing Side Bend Pose

Create the kavana (*intention*):

Visualize expanding your inner energy as you softly move your body from side to side and awaken the divine within. The side bend brings balance to the entire body by lengthening the abdominal muscles, hips, thigh muscles, and spine.

Directions into the pose:

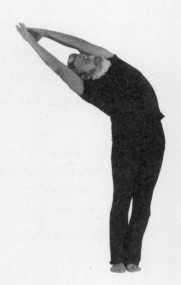

1. Come into Mountain Pose. Feel the lift of your lower body while you draw your tailbone down.

2. Keeping your hips neutral and shoulders away from your ears, inhale and extend your arms up toward the sky, palms facing one another.

3. Gently stretch your arms toward the left, keeping your shoulder blades reaching down and your hips neutral, always allowing some space at your left waist, and keeping your right shoulder back.

4. Breathe into your right side, allowing your breath to travel through the spaces between your ribs, always equally pressing your feet down.

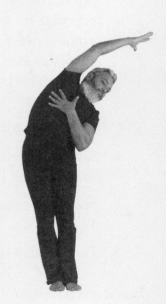

5. Place your opposite hand onto your heart and softly breathe into it.

6. After a few breaths, come back to neutral, and experiment with the pose on the other side.

Health and benefits:

- Lengthens the abdominals, hips, and thighs
- Creates flexibility in the spine
- Stretches the muscles between the ribs
- Opens the lungs and rib cage
- Improves breathing

Side Plank Variation

Create the kavana (*intention*):

Visualize that you are a carrier of light, and the deeper you draw inward, the further you share your light. Side Plank strengthens your arms and wrists as you work your balance.

Directions into the pose:

1. Start in Plank Pose, stacking your shoulders above your wrists.

2. Move away from the Earth by lifting the back of your heart and lungs. You will feel more space in your back and more activity in your arms, always keeping a small bending motion in your elbows.

3. Come to the outer edge of your left foot, bringing your right foot flat on the Earth, at the level of your hips. Using the balance of your three foundations (feet and hand), start to lengthen your right arm up to the sky, and then above your head.

4. If you want to evolve into the pose, into your next exhale, stack your right leg fully on top of the left. Feel a strong connection with your left arm into the Earth, and keep your shoulder blades drawn into your back.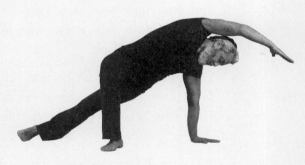

5. Lift your hips away from the Earth, allowing your upper ribs to open toward the sky and taking the shape of an arc.

6. Take a few breaths here. The more you connect to your foundation, the more you can expand your openness.

7. Smoothly come into Downward Dog, before coming back into Plank Pose.

8. Do the other side.

Health and benefits:

*   Strengthens and stretches the arms, wrists, legs, and belly

*   Improves balance

Wild Thing

Create the kavana (*intention*):

Imagine your inner light spreading through your entire body as you connect to the Earth, sky, and energy surrounding you. The Wild Thing is energetic and playful, and builds balance and core strength as you reveal your inner heart and grace through the pose.

Directions into the pose:

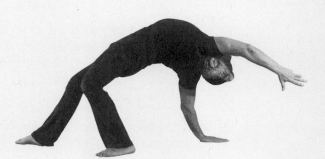

1. Start in Downward Dog, staying for a good five breaths to connect to your roots.

2. Come into Side Plank on your right side.

3. Step your left foot behind you, keeping your right leg straight, and pushing your hips up and away from the Earth.

4. Scoop your tailbone and use your legs to keep lifting your hips.

5. Curl your head back, lift the left side of your body, and extend your left arm over your head, keeping your shoulder blades reaching down toward your hips.

6. From your roots, deepen your side bend into a beautiful and graceful backbend.

7. After a few breaths, release, and step back into Downward Dog. Switch sides.

Health and benefits:

- Stretches the chest, shoulders, hip flexors, and front of the legs
- Opens the heart and throat
- Strengthens the arms, shoulders, and upper back
- Invigorates the body and mind

CHAPTER 21

SHIN: Inner Peace

Pose: Wide-Legged Forward Bend

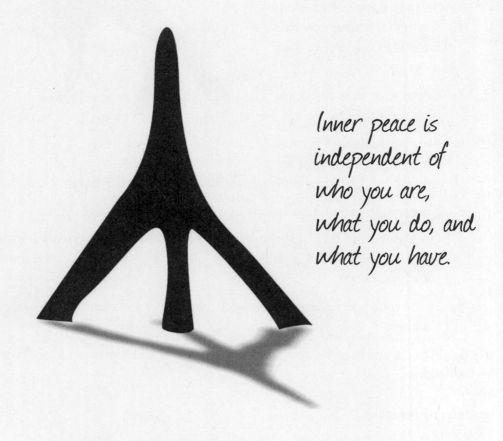

Inner peace is independent of who you are, what you do, and what you have.

The *Shin* corresponds to the combined English letters *SH* and has a numerical value of 300.

Soul

Shin: Shai Shel Shalom Osin Ba'Olam Hazeh. "Peace is a precious gift we can offer to this world."

—Akivah

The Maggid of Mezeritch, a great Hassidic master, was once asked by his students, "How could anyone reach the level of inner peace discussed in *The Talmud* (*Brachot*), that 'a person is required to bless the Creator with the same fervor for the bad as he would bless for the good experiences in life'?" The Maggid told them to go to his student Reb Zusha for the answer.

They went to the house of Reb Zusha. They could not help but notice how tattered his clothes were, and still his face radiated light. He lived in a small apartment with his family. During the day, the house was a living room and dining room where they would eat and Reb Zusha would study the secrets with students. They saw that there was very little food and that everyone in his family was sharing small portions of bread. At night, the room was transformed into a large bedroom for the entire family. Reb Zusha could not even afford a bed, so he would sleep on the wooden bench used during the day for meals and study.

The students were stunned, and certain that their question was going to be answered. They told Reb Zusha that the Maggid had sent them to him to receive the answer to the question in *The Talmud*, "How can anyone bless the Creator for the bad with the same fervor as he would for the good?" He pondered, closed his eyes, and looked inward. Reb Zusha was surprised that the Maggid had sent them to him, and advised them to go find a person who was suffering in order to find the answer. Reb Zusha told them that he was at peace because he never experienced anything bad in his entire life. How could he answer such a question?

As the students left, they realized that their question had been answered. Not everyone lives the hard life of Reb Zusha, but we can all relate to the struggle we must go through to find peace. Some people seem to find it easily, while others labor each day in search of it. No matter how hard it may be to reach peace, it is an option most of us strive for.

Peace can be pursued in a way that is internal or external. Internal peace is what we look for inside ourselves as we draw into our depth through prayer, meditation, devotion, and awareness. External peace has to do with our physical lives, how we live materially, what we value, and where we place our priorities. Both are important, but the advantage of searching for internal peace is that it will be more powerful than any other form of happiness. Inner *shalom* exists independent of who you are, what you do, or what you have. It is, simply, what is inside of you beyond the layers of skin, flesh, and bones. The external forms of peace may come and go and often change, and will always be conditional on external circumstances. Even internal peace can be conditional if it becomes dependent upon circumstances outside of us.

Inner peace occurs when we are busy with opposites and yet have the vision to see them flowing together. It is experienced when the soul sees its mission through the body, and united, the body and soul do their part on Earth as one. Internally, peace is felt in our mind and heart. Thoughts and feelings have power over us. They can shape and mold us to be a certain type of person. If, however, they are not in harmony, they become uncontrollable and cause fear and judgment.

The mind has an influence that can bring us either to something in the past or to somewhere that has not yet happened. Being in the present moment removes these doubtful thoughts. We cannot change something that has already occurred, so how do we benefit from worrying about it? Similarly, worrying about something that potentially could or could not happen is useless. Instead, we need to cultivate the present moment through stillness, faith, and trust in the universe that the path to inner peace can be revealed through us.

Trust and faith in the Creator are things that we must nurture. Faith allows us to see peace as a goal to reach for. Jewish homes customarily place a mezuzah on the right side of the doorpost with a letter *Shin* engraved on its cover to remind us that our paths and experiences can be blessings for *shalom*, "peace." Inside the mezuzah case is the most sacred prayer in Judaism, the Shema Yisrael, which speaks about the Creator being our empowerment and oneness in all our experiences. Because the Creator exists within, what we experience through our challenges is the universe acting within to attain oneness. Unlike singularity, which implies uniqueness, oneness is togetherness achieved by combining the many to becoming one. If we focus on what we have in common instead of what makes us different, we can achieve peace among ourselves. Peace is cultivated in relationships that have honor and respect. If we see the wisdom in our differences, then we will be at peace with the knowledge that each of us can help complete and benefit the other.

Peace will not be found if we only care for ourselves. We cannot expect to have true harmony if our whole motivation is self-consuming and is only about serving our own needs and desires. Kindness, compassion, and understanding toward each other are the keys that open the door to real peace. When we care for each other, positivity will stem from this bond and reinforce our feelings of inner peace.

When the heart is faced with challenges, it will express feelings. The mind will fill the brain with ongoing thoughts. Often these thoughts cause confusion as we become emotional about people and situations. In reality, our relationships and situations will be empowered by the way we see them. If we see the whole picture of ourselves and think positively, we will realize that the challenges we are going through are all part of the same goal of finding wholeness in our pursuit of peace.

If we do not challenge our thoughts to see through to serenity, we will not find wholeness, because we live by accepting the negative ones as a permanent part of us. They will start to influence our beliefs and convictions and eventually redefine who we are. But if we become positive, optimistic, kind, and compassionate instead, then they will be the fuel of our reactions and actions.

The Alter Rebbe (author of the *Tanya*) teaches that we can control our thoughts and prevent them from turning negative by awakening the intelligence of the heart. It may be difficult and almost impossible to change every thought, feeling, and emotion. What we can do is change the relationship between the heart and mind.

When a negative thought comes to mind, we need to free ourselves from it by drawing into the wisdom of our emotions. When we have a positive one, we need to cultivate its intelligence and create *kavana*, deep intentions from the heart, so the wisdom of the heart leads us into harmony.

This wisdom tells us that our true self can be different from our thoughts. The Alter Rebbe defines thoughts as an outer garment of the soul. Inwardly, our genuine state is to be at peace. However, the mind, an exterior layer, can say otherwise. Like clothes, thoughts are not permanent, and so we must not give them more importance than required. They come and go, and depending on what we saw, felt, heard, or experienced, they will affect how we live. The *Shin* teaches us that the heart's warmth—made of love, compassion, and understanding—forms the fire of *shalom*, known as *shalhevet*, symbolized by its three lines coming together at one root. We can choose to change our thoughts for the good so they resemble the way we really feel internally.

For our practice of yoga to be from the essence, we need to create within us an opening for *shalom* so there is a flow between our breath and our movement. I often begin my practice by warming the body with Salutations that include the Hebrew letters that spell *shalom* by posturing into the letter *Shin* variations, along with the letters *Lamed* for an open heart, *Vav* for alignment, and *Mem* for space, to connect the body and soul with the energy of *shalom*.

The secret of *shalom* is found in its syllables. The *sha* relates to the *neshama*, "soul"; the *la* sound to the *lev*, "heart"; and the *om* to the potential of body (*om* in Hebrew means "physical strength"). When searching for *shalom*, we need to ignite the light of our soul, nurture and warm the heart, and illuminate the body. While the soul searches for purpose, the body can be in one place and the heart elsewhere. With *shalom*, we can find genuine harmony among the three so peace becomes real for us in the soul, heart, and body.

Having inner peace can be as easy as letting go of what holds us back from being internally free. Inner silence is important to peace and can be felt by simply sitting on a park bench enjoying the sun shining, birds singing, and the magnificent scenery.

The Letter

The letter *Shin* has the sound of "shhh," which we often say when we want some quiet. Silence is what we look for in our search for peace. When we are internally still, our senses become more open and less distracted by our mental and emotional chatter. We listen in order to take in, to be more aware, to learn and to teach, and to be interested in and care for those around us. If you want to hear what someone is saying, listen carefully to their words as you may hear their soul talking. We were created with two ears and only one mouth to remind us that if we want to have inner peace, we need to do more listening than talking. Attentiveness permits us to evaluate our words and speak from the heart to make sure that we are speaking with sensitivity and understanding. We should strive to always talk softly, honestly, and with consideration for others so our words will be received peacefully. Inner silence is essential to our inner peace, and can be achieved through breathing, meditation, visualization, and more.

The search for *shalom* is an option we have and should not be chosen for a fleeting moment, but a continuous pursuit. Grow now from your inspiration to inner peace. Seize each moment that follows as an opportunity to renew yourself with the light, simplicity, acceptance, and hope of *shalom*.

Breath: Energetic Shape and Intention

The kavanas of the Shin are feelings of peace, humility, serenity, selflessness, and introversion. The intention is also acceptance, kindness, love, compassion, and understanding.

The three pillars of the letter *Shin* are formed though the legs and the torso folding forward to be in line with the feet. The symbolism is that inner peace is achieved when the mind, heart, and body come together in harmony. The inhale is at the extension of the spine while creating space in the body. The inhale is also the lifting of the heart, as you take in the energy of *shalom* and connect to its source. The exhale is the folding of the body to the Earth and the drawing of the heart into the depths of yourself.

In the Wide-Legged Forward Bend with a Twist, your breath emerges from your core as you twist deeply to each direction. On an inhale, press your hand to the floor to create rootedness. On an exhale, bring your navel in deeper to enhance your twist.

In the Wide-Angle Seated Forward Bend, you connect to the Earth by letting go and pressing down on your legs, feeling every muscle melting and softly contracting your muscles. On an inhale, lengthen and expand your upper body. On an exhale, release your upper body to the Earth.

In the variation of opening to the side, the inhale is at opening your front body to the side and the expansion of your lungs. The exhale is at the settling down and maintaining the pose as you go deeper into the openness.

Body

Poses:

Wide-Legged Forward Bend

Wide-Legged Forward Bend with a Twist

Wide-Angle Seated Forward Bend

Wide-Legged Forward Bend

Create the kavana (*intention*):

See your mind being free of any thought as you lengthen to the foundations of your heart. The Wide-Legged Forward Bend stretches the hamstrings, inner and outer legs, and spine and calms the mind.

Directions into the pose:

1. Stand in Mountain Pose. Separate your feet about three to four feet apart. Keep the outer edges of your feet parallel to the edges of the mat, pressing them into the mat, and feel your inner arches lift away from the Earth.

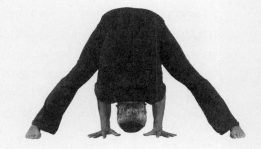

2. Bring your hands to your hips and engage your thigh muscles. While inhaling, lengthen the front of your upper body.

3. On your next exhale, keep that length, and fold over your hips. Release your hands to the floor at the width of your shoulders, pressing firmly and keeping a long upper body parallel to the floor.

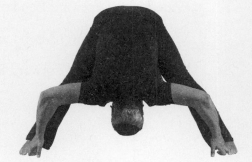

4. To go further, reach out and grab with your peace fingers for your big toe on each foot.

5. Envision holding on to your big toes as a reminder to embrace *shalom*, peace and serenity.

6. Take a few breaths here, focusing on the lengthening of your legs, spine, and arms.

7. Exhale, go deeper inside, and feel your *shalom*.

8. Slowly start walking your hands backward until you reach the space between your feet.

9. Keep your sternum long, and fold a little bit more, allowing your elbows to bend to the side, keeping a nice attraction between your arms, lifting your sitting bones toward the sky, and lengthening the backs of your legs. The crown of your head will reach toward the Earth, while your shoulder blades reach toward your hips.

10. Take a few breaths here, and to come out of the pose, walk your hands forward, bringing your upper body parallel to the floor again.

11. Bring your hands to your hips, engage your center, and lift your upper body.

12. Bring your feet together and return to Mountain Pose.

Health and benefits:

- Strengthens and stretches the inner legs, backs of the legs, and spine
- Tones the abdominal organs
- Calms the brain
- Relieves mild backache

Wide-Legged Forward Bend with a Twist

Create the kavana (intention):

Imagine that by twisting into the pose, you are going deeper into your essence and freeing your heart to each side.

Directions into the pose:

1. Follow the instructions for the Wide-Legged Forward Bend.

2. Bring your left hand to the floor between your feet, directly under your chest.

3. Inhale and lengthen your spine.

4. On the exhale, twist to the right, bringing your right hand to your sacrum to keep your hips square and neutral.

5. Stay here for a few breaths.

6. To go further, inhale, and stretch your right arm up toward the sky, keeping your hips neutral and twisting through your torso.

7. Gaze up toward your right thumb and visualize your body being the vehicle of peace.

8. Take a few deep breaths, focusing on your rootedness and openness.

9. Release on an exhale, and do the other side.

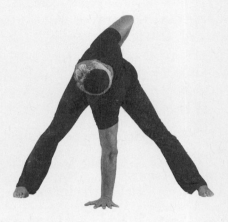

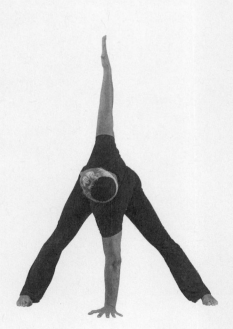

Health and benefits:

- Stretches the hamstrings, calves, hips, lower back, and spine
- Stretches and strengthens the upper back and shoulders
- Opens the hips
- Calms the brain
- Detoxifies the digestive organs
- Soothes the mind
- Improves full-body coordination

Wide-Angle Seated Forward Bend

Create the kavana *(intention):*

Softly settle your heart into the Earth and allow the moment to be your inspiration for *shalom*. The Wide-Angle Seated Forward Bend is a seated pose that stretches the legs and spine deeply and quiets the mind of stress.

Directions into the pose:

1. Sit in Staff Pose, and open your legs to an angle of about ninety degrees. Feel the pressing down of your sitting bones into the Earth.

2. Make sure your knees are always pointing up. Press your heels into the Earth.

3. On your next inhale, keeping your sternum long, bring your hands to the floor in front of you, shoulder-width apart.

4. Press your hands with your fingers wide open into the Earth, and continue widening your chest, on every exhale drawing your shoulder blades down.

5. Slowly walk your hands forward, and on every exhale, deepen your forward bend, with your heart, still, soft, open, and reaching toward the Earth.

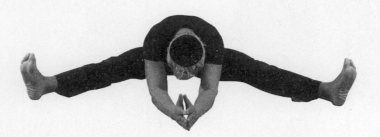

Health and benefits:

- Opens the hips while stretching out the entire back of the body
- Stretches the insides of the legs
- Stimulates the abdominal organs
- Strengthens the spine
- Calms the brain

CHAPTER 22

TAV: Passion

Pose: The Cat

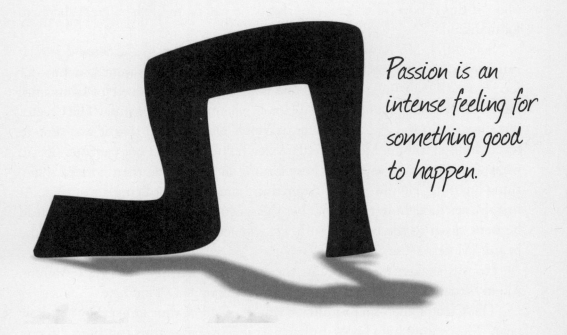

Passion is an intense feeling for something good to happen.

The *Tav* corresponds to the letter *T* and has a numerical value of 400.

Soul

Tav: Ta'avato She-Hu Mit-aveh Bechol Yom. "Sacred passion is cultivated each day."

—Akivah

One day while Moses was strolling in the desert of Sinai with his herd of sheep, one small sheep ran away from the flock. Moses followed the little sheep to a pond of water. He saw that the sheep wanted to drink water and had only run away because she was thirsty. He embraced her with much love, picked her up on his shoulders, and carried her back to the flock. The Creator saw this and said, "If this is how Moses cares for sheep, he will certainly be a great shepherd for mankind!"

Soon after, Moses was again strolling with his sheep in the Sinai desert. It was late in the afternoon, and his sheep were hungry. Moses went searching for food but could not find pasture ground for the sheep. He walked for hours until he reached a small mountain called Horeb, where he found pasture. The Creator saw once again the great character in Moses, and decided that it was time to reveal himself to him. Moses heard a voice talking, but did not pay attention to what was being said, as he was busy feeding his sheep. He then noticed something amazing. He saw a bush covered in flames but not being consumed. At first, Moses thought to turn away, but the spectacle was too powerful, so instead he went closer to the burning bush. He listened to the voice, and this time he heard, "Moses! Moses!"

He was shaken to his core as the voice sounded like his father Amram, whom he had not seen for years. He humbly responded, "I am here!"

The Creator then said to him, "I am the God of your father. Do not draw near." Moses wore high boots in shepherd style to protect his feet from difficult paths and bodies of water in the wilderness. The Creator then said to him, "Take off your shoes, because the place upon which you stand is sacred soil" (Exodus 3:1-5).

There is so much to learn from this story. When the Creator spoke to the ancestors, Adam, Eve, Noah, and Abraham, the first conversations were always direct. But when it came to Moses, the greatest leader of the Bible, the Creator chose to speak with him from a bush. Why?

Clearly the Creator wanted to reveal to Moses a wisdom about the burning bush that would apply to him and to anyone he would teach.

Let us look at the story backward. Before approaching the burning bush, Moses needed to know that he was standing on sacred soil. The Creator was telling Moses that wherever we are standing in life, we can cultivate the sacred in the soil underneath us and experience a higher awakening.

To unleash the energy of our sacred soil, we need to *Shal Ne'alecha*, "Take off our shoes," meaning remove the layers and restrictions that prevent us from shining out. *Ne'alecha* also means "locks," and refers to unlocking your heart so that your true self can be revealed. We often form unnecessary knots in our hearts because of deceptions, broken love, and pain. To unlock the heart, we need to draw into the essence and nurture it.

The bush is our heart. Like a bush, there can be thorns blocking us from entering into the essence of our heart. Inside the bush is an energy that can blossom flowers and bear fruits. To cultivate the heart, there needs to be a desire to rise above and ignite the fire within.

The Letter

The letter *Tav* in Hebrew means "passion." Passion is a feeling of a strong and intense emotion for something to happen. It is often an inexplicable desire to experience certain conditions that bring joy.

Passion becomes our guide as we grow deeply into inspiration. If we see that there is hope and good for others in what we do, then our passion will become our own good and deep breath.

When we are passionate, we draw into our higher self by kindling a fire of enthusiasm in our heart to see something happen. The heart then begins to move upward like flames yearning to rise higher into the eternal flame and connect with our source. The power of passion is that its fire does not consume the bush, the body of life that carries it.

As much as we rise higher into the fire of our passions, we should remain connected to the realities of our life so everything about us is inspired and elevated by our passions. If our passions, however, separate us from the people that matter in our life, they will consume our heart, and we will no longer be connected to the eternal light.

A revered teacher, once guiding a meditation for his students, lit several candles and said, "Listen to what the flames are saying." Does a flame talk or make a sound? What about a soul; when it rises, does it make a sound?

The soul, like a flame, also rises upward as if to detach itself from its body and be united with the eternal flame. Like a flame, the soul craves to rise from its material trappings and be free from the restrictions of life, to reunite with its source. The soul wants to do its part in the body and fulfill its mission on Earth to be a bringer of light. To do so, the flame-soul within must be nurtured.

For the soul's light to be revealed, there must be oil in the heart to feel its warmth, clarity in the mind to meditate on its greatness, and a body with a desire to carry it, experience it, and share its radiance with others.

It is not the flame nor the soul that makes the sound. These rise in stillness as they absorb and lose themselves into the eternal light. Rather, the noise comes from the physical interaction between the oil of the heart and wick of the mind, held together by the body that brings them together to make a fire. Similarly, the noise that comes from the interaction of the body and soul comes from the fire of the heart born through passion.

The burning bush teaches us that the fire of the heart is not something that exists for itself. Instead, it is to motivate and inspire us to illuminate our surroundings. Similar to a flame that can ignite a thousand other candles and never lose its strength, so too a burning fire in the heart has the power to affect so much around us.

The secret of the fire in the heart is that it is more powerful than the greatest darkness. No matter how dark it may be, a fire in the heart will always shine brightly if it is cultivated. Its peaceful, silent, and soothing glow can influence any person or situation.

Each day is an opportunity to create such a powerful light in our life, whether it is at work, at home, or socially. When the mind wanders, it is time to allow the heart to lead the way to warm up our path and overcome our challenges without conflict that ignites the flame of peace we desperately require.

The sages ask, "How do we cultivate the heart?" The answer they give is through the service of *tefillah*, the Hebrew word translated as "prayer," which begins with the letter *Tav*.

In English, "prayer" derives from the Latin *precare*, which suggests to beg or beseech. *Tefillah* is much more than that. *Tefillah* is the work of creating a burning bush in the heart. By cultivating through *tefillah*, we create passion by connecting deeply to our inner self in order to connect to the universe.

Unlike prayer, *tefillah* is doing something powerful for ourselves. By drawing into our heart, we are tapping into a great reservoir of strength and enthusiasm concealed inside, waiting to be revealed. By expressing with passion what is in our heart, we heal ourselves and others. By listening to what we are praying for, we examine who we are and confront our fears and worries. Only then does our potential express itself. The Creator does not need to hear our prayers to know what is in our heart. He knows well what we are lacking and what our wishes are—to live a better life. But we need *tefillah* in order to listen to our inner voice and become aware of what we are asking for. What do we pray for? Do we pray only for ourselves, or do we also pray for others? Are our prayers only about material things, or are they also about our spirit?

For passion to be powerful and lasting, it must stem from our heart. From the heart, we extend our passion to our thoughts and influence our way of thinking, speaking, and listening. When the head has been touched by a warm heart, then our actions also begin to be influenced by the passion that comes from a warm heart.

Find passion in your life and use it to reach deeply into yourself. Keep in mind that today's achievement is tomorrow's starting point. Tomorrow's fulfillment will then be the following day's beginning, and so on. Passion can grow for a long time and become natural if we nourish it, care for it, and let it flourish.

Breath: Energetic Shape and Intention

The kavanas *of the Tav are feelings of passion, desire, and will. It is the opening of your heart to feelings of love, compassion, and soulfulness.*

The shape of the letter *Tav* is assumed by opening the heart to experiencing deeper feelings. We can shape into it by doing the Table Top and Cat Poses. Because it is the letter for passion, when we move into its shape, we look inward into the heart by coiling our spine, or by arching the lower back, and we open our heart in order to reveal this passion externally.

In the Table Top Pose, you deeply connect to the subtle movement of your spine. The inhale focuses on the opening and lengthening of the front of the spine, and the exhale focuses on the back of the spine. At the end of your inhalation you can stay, allowing a moment with your full lungs, and then exhale fully to round the back. You can lengthen the pose by staying in it with your lungs empty. This process will lengthen the pose and create more awareness of the impact of your breath on your organs and movements.

In the Cat Pose variation, you combine the breath with the balancing sensation, using your core and centering on each exhale to maintain the balance, while the inhale adds more length from your fingers to your heel. Your breath in this pose helps relieve stress, fatigue, and tension.

The *Tav*, as in Dolphin Pose, presses the forearms upon the Earth as a symbol that if your passions are cultivated like seeds planted in the ground, then they will grow positively. Dolphin Pose is demanding on the shoulders and brings a great awareness of the tightness you might feel in this part of the body. The breath will be here to release that tension. You can learn to breathe into your whole upper back, widening, creating space, and allowing the breath to have an intention of deep release.

You will probably need to use your breath to focus on your strength, at the level of your arms and shoulders. Let it flow, following the rhythm of the inhale and exhale, expansion and contraction, space and rootedness.

Passion will begin when you experience a powerful feeling for something or someone that creates a deep interest inside of you. The degree of your passion will depend upon the level of your personal involvement in the activity that makes you excited. The more you give of yourself, the more you let go of your limitations, worries, and anxieties and the more fully will your passion be realized, the more will your soul be given expression.

In your yoga practice, it is the flow you create when you move your body with rhythm and breath that leads you into grace and calm. Your postures become peaceful flames, striving to reach for the sky and yet remaining connected to the Earth. Your breath is therefore the oxygen of your inner candle, moving the flame inside upward, softly and smoothly.

Body

Poses:

Table Top Pose

Cat Pose Variation: Table Pose with Extended Arm

Dolphin Pose

Table Top Pose

Create the kavana (*intention*):

Focus on the line of energy you create stretching from your heart and into your hands and toes as you connect to the Earth.

Directions into the Pose:

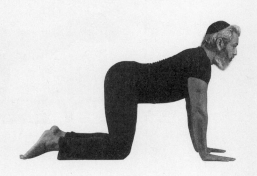

1. Come to your hands and knees in a table-top position. Make sure your knees are directly under your hips and your wrists, elbows, and shoulders in line.

2. Take the time to lengthen your spine, draw in your navel, and feel your breath from your sitting bones to the crown of your head.

3. On your next exhale, round your spine toward the ceiling, and gently bring your chin in and tailbone down.

4. On the next inhalation, lift your sitting bones up toward the sky, and open your heart and chest. Gaze forward.

5. Use the next few breaths to go from one pose to the other, inhaling, opening your heart, and exhaling, bringing everything in. Make sure to open your fingers wide, pressing into the floor at the base of your fingers.

6. After ten to fifteen repetitions, come back to the neutral table-top position.

Health and benefits:

- Stretches the back, torso, and neck
- Stretches the shoulders, chest, and abdominal muscles
- Provides a gentle massage to the spine and belly organs
- Relieves stress

Cat Pose Variation: Table Pose with Extended Arm

Create the kavana (*intention*):

Envision that as you coil your spine, you are drawing deeper into your heart and reaching for your essence.

Directions into the pose:

1. Start on your hands and knees, with your hands directly under your shoulders and your knees directly under your hips (in Table Top Pose).

2. Gaze at a point between your palms.

3. Draw your navel up to your spine, keeping your back neutral.

4. Extend your right leg backward, parallel to the floor.

5. With your abdominal muscles engaged, extend your left arm forward, keeping it at the level of your shoulder.

6. Hold for a few breaths, feeling the length of your whole body and connecting through your midline.

7. Bring your knee and arm down and do the pose on the other side.

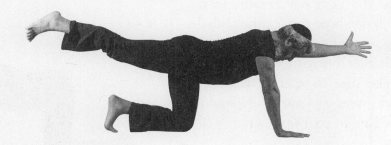

Health and benefits:

- Strengthens the abdominals and lower back
- Brings flexibility to the spine, shoulders, and hips
- Stretches the torso
- Improves focus, coordination, and physical equilibrium

Dolphin Pose

Create the kavana (*intention*):

Envision connecting to the energy of the Earth with your arms and fingers spread out as you lengthen your heart forward.

Directions into the pose:

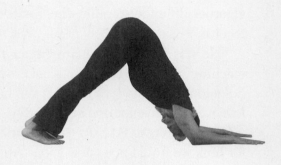

1. Start in Table Top Pose, with your knees directly under your hips.

2. Bring your forearms to the floor, keeping them parallel to one another, and making sure that your elbows are directly under your shoulders. Keep a deep rootedness with your forearms on the Earth.

3. Tuck your toes, and on your exhalation, lift your knees away from the floor.

4. Press strongly into the Earth and bring your sitting bones up and back. You can walk your feet in if there is openness in your shoulders. Continuously lengthen up and back, pressing your heels down and keeping the length in your spine and the backs of your legs.

5. Continue actively pressing your forearms into the Earth, with your shoulder blades sliding down toward your hips.

6. Hold your head between the upper arms, moving away from the floor.

7. Stay for a few breaths, and then release your knees down to the floor on an exhale.

Health and benefits:

- Calms the brain, and relieves stress and mild depression
- Strengthens the arms and legs
- Stretches the shoulders, hamstrings, and calves
- Relieves headache, insomnia, back pain, and fatigue

A FINAL NOTE

Each chapter began with a little inspiring teaching from Akivah, a simple man who lived during the end of the first century and the beginning of the second. He is one of the most revered Jewish sages of all time. *The Talmud* compares his greatness in understanding the Torah to Moses, the highest honor a person can receive.

He was loved by so many because he spent so much time embodying and teaching about love. Akivah once said that if the Torah is holy, then King Solomon's book *Song of Songs* is the holy of holies because it is about the great love we can have for one another.

It is thanks to Akivah that we understand the Hebrew letters. If it were not for him, we would not know about Abraham's *Sefer Yetsirah, The Book of Shapes*. He taught us about the meaning of the letters, their unique shapes, and their secrets in Kabalah. Akivah is the author of *Midrash, Otiot d'Rabbi Akivah*, a small manuscript written almost as a personal diary to share the wisdom he had gathered on Hebrew letters, which I have quoted throughout this book at the beginning of each chapter.

His background, however, was nothing in comparison to what he would become. As a child, Akivah struggled to be accepted by society. He was a child of converts and a descendant of Sisera, an evil commander who persecuted the Jewish people during the days of the prophetess Deborah.

No one paid him much attention. He grew up as a shepherd and did not learn how to read or write until middle age. Rachel, the daughter of his wealthy master, Kalba, fell in love with him due to his humility and humanity. Although he was a poor shepherd who spent his days caring for her father's herd of sheep, she saw in him a great shepherd who would one day lead thousands of people. She proposed to marry him if he would dedicate time to study the Torah. He loved her so much that he accepted, not knowing how he would go about it.

When his master heard about the secret marriage, he was angered and fired Akivah, kicking his daughter out of his house and promising that he would never help her if she stayed married to the illiterate man. Although she then had to live in difficult poverty, Rachel loved Akivah very much and continued to envision that one day he would reach his greatest potential.

Still, Akivah had sadness in his heart, realizing that he was a grown man incapable of learning because he could not read. He continued to be a shepherd, but his thirst for drinking from the well of Torah's wisdom had grown more painful.

One day, while shepherding, he took a different path. He saw a rock underneath a well that was soft on the outside and deep on the inside, as it had hollow spaces carved into it. He inquired about the rock that had made an impression on him, and was told by other shepherds that the hollow spaces in the rock were caused by the slow persistent dripping of water that came from the well. The softening of the rock's surface was due to water drops softly splashing onto the surface of the rock and spreading itself onto it.

Akiva was enlightened. For the first time, he finally understood what he had to do. He thought to himself: *If a rock, which is hard, can be dug deeply into by the slow and persistent movement of water, then certainly my brain can be opened if I begin to learn drop by drop. If a rock can be softened by the gentle spreading of water on its surface, then my heart, too, can be soothed by the slow and subtle movement of understanding.*

Then, at the age of forty, he began attending kindergarten with his infant children. He learned from the drops of water that fell on the rock that if he wanted to learn Torah, he had to start from the very beginning through the Hebrew letters, the first drops of wisdom children are taught before learning the Torah.

He was laughed at and ridiculed for spending his time with children. Still this did not discourage Akivah. His daily mantra was, "If a rock can be penetrated, then I can be deepened. If a rock can be softened, then I can be softened."

He continued to persevere in understanding the Hebrew letters, how they formed ideas, and their unique shapes and meanings. With the encouragement of his wife, Rachel, he studied for the next twenty-four years away from home. Rachel supported Akivah as she saw that he was slowly becoming the vision she had in him of being a shepherd of mankind. When he finally returned home, he was accompanied by twenty-four thousand students (one thousand for each year he studied), who came with him to honor Rachel for what he had become thanks to her.

~~~~~~~~~~~~~~~~~~~~~~~~~~~~~

I share the story of Akivah because he represents each of us in our struggle to reach our potential. We often feel poor in the qualities we think we need to have in order to be somewhere we want to be. Sometimes the dream we have of ourselves seems to be at a far distance, when really it is very close. Akivah came from circumstances that normally prevent a person from moving forward. Yet because of his immense spirit, he was able to transform himself to be his best at the most difficult moments of his life. The story of Akivah reminds us that it is never too late to fulfill our dreams, to be our visions, and to live the full, happy life we desire.

This book should be viewed as the drops of water Akivah saw dripping on the rock, reminding you that step by step, you can embrace your dreams if you are willing to change your perception.

Whatever level your challenges may take you to, whether they affect you externally or internally, remember: "If a rock can be penetrated, then I can be deepened. If a rock can be softened, then I can be softened!"

Akivah's story is symbolic of what patience and slow drops of wisdom can do to soften our body and open our heart and mind.

When we start to visualize more positively and surround ourselves with love, everything becomes possible. The body is constantly carrying messages, and if we commit to irrigating the soil of the mind and heart, then these messages grow into positiveness. Positiveness begins with how you see yourself: your body as a temple, your heart as an altar, and your mind as an offering. When you start to consider yourself as sacred, then you have made space for the sacredness of the soul to be revealed, to soften, to penetrate, and to shine through you.

The moment could be now to make a change in the way you see your body and soul connection and purpose in life. You are the Creator's beautiful gift to life.

Trust in the Creator who trusts in you.

Know that it is never too late to make a change.

Never stop learning, teaching, or sharing.

Grow. Be inspired. Believe in yourself.

Do not allow fear to limit you.

Open your heart to take in and give back.

I wrote this book as if I were talking to you. Throughout the pages, I reflect on my personal life and stories that inspired me. Know that my intention was to share with you all that we have in common.

Embody the sacred letters. Shape into them and connect to their energy. Meditate on their meaning as a daily practice and grow from these drops.

ACKNOWLEDGMENTS

Thank you:

To the Creator for believing in us.

To the ancestors, sages, and mystics, your voices whisper throughout the pages.

If the soul had one honor to give, it would be to the body who carried it throughout its journey.

To my beloved Karen, who I am forever grateful for.

To the fruits that came from our tree: Shamai, Geoulah, Maayan, Tsemach, Tanya, Neshama, Shalom, and Shimon. Your spirit embraces me. Love you!

To my sister, Michal, and to my Ima: you are always in my heart. To my brother Eric: thank you from my heart for everything you do! To my dad in heaven; I feel you each day!

I would like to thank some special people who made this book possible: my agent Ava Taylor of YAMA Talent, Gary Rosen of RLR, and Scott Gould, my book agent. I salute New Harbinger and, particularly, Katie Parr and Heather Garnos as well as Gretel Hakanson for copyediting the entire book and making sure it is at its best. Jennifer Buergermeister for reviewing the book at its initial state and for giving me insightful suggestions. Divvy Ahronheim for being by my side until the finish, helping in the editing and organization of the book. I am proud of my son Shamai for researching sources of many ancient teachings. Reb Greenglass obm, and Reb Meir Abehsera obm: mentors. Thank you for your inspiration and guidance. R. Zalman Kaplan: our learning together on the breath according to Kabalah and your wise advice has helped me tremendously in writing this book. R. Moshe New, thank you for your encouragement. David Puterman, Eli BenDavid, Ariel Cozocaru, Dubi Dahan, Rocking Rabbi, Alain Malka, and Haim Sherff, your friendship and support each one of you in your own unique way is very appreciated. To author and meditation teacher Lorin Roche, thank you for sharing your knowledge about the historical connection of the Jews with India. To the brothers at the House of Love, I cherish our deep bonds cultivated through prayer and meditation. Saadia Elhadad for sharing R. Nachman's teachings and Ras Daveed for introducing me to Abulafia's Kabbalah.

My learning colleagues Rabbis Naftali Perlstein and Yankee Feder: the mysteries would not be as deep without you.

I extend gratitude to my executive producer, Moses Znaimer, for realizing the vision of Kabalah Yoga into a daily TV show across Canada. Zalman Glassner for putting your best imagination into the development of Kabalah Yoga. Ofer Alduby for your incredible eye in the filming of the videos. Shalom Serraf for the great photography of the poses.

Yoga teachers that inspired me throughout the years: Karen Claffey, Dharma Mittra, Hart Lazer, Amy Weintraub, Michele Bohbot, and Moses Love: thank you for sharing your wisdom on yoga.

Thank you to all the yoga teachers and students I have met on the path.

To Shiva Rea: thank you for opening your heart and sharing so much from deep inside. Eternal gratitude to you. To my spiritual brother Demetrios Velisarius, your energy has inspired me. To the Prana Vinyasa tribe: thank you for being an awesome family.

ENDNOTES

1   Rabbi Akivah ben Yosef, *Midrash, Otiot d'Rabbi Akivah* (Jerusalem: Yarid Hasefarim, 1999).

2   Rabbi Schneur Zalman, *Torah Or* (New York: "Kehot" Publication Society, 1999); Yakov Kouli, *Yalkut Me'am Lo'ez* (Israel: Samuel, 1967); and *Sages of the Talmud Sanhedrin* (New York: Mesorah Publications Ltd., 2002).

3   Stefan G. Hofman, Paul Grossman, and Devon E. Hinton, "Loving-Kindness and Compassion Meditation: Potential for Psychological Interventions," *Clinical Psychology Review* 31 (2011). doi: 10.1016/j.cpr.2011.07.003; and Barbara L. Fredrickson, Michael A. Cohn, Kimberly A. Coffey, Jolynn Pek, and Sandra M. Finkel, "Open Hearts Build Lives: Positive Emotions, Induced Through Loving-Kindness Meditation, Build Consequential Personal Resources," *Journal of Personality and Social Psychology* 95 (2008). doi: 10.1037/a0013262.

4   Rabbi Chaim Miller, *Genesis, 1:1, The Gutnick Edition* (New York: Kol Menachem, 2008). Schneur Zalman, *Sages, Morning Liturgy, Tehillat Hashem*, trans. Nissan Mangel (New York: Merkos L'nyonei Chinuch, 2013).

5   Rabbi M. M. Schneerson, *Hayom Yom, "From Day to Day"* (New York: Otzar Hachassidim Lubavitch, 1988).

6   Schneur Zalman of Liadi [the Alter Rebbe], *Tanya* (New York: Kehot Publication Society, 1984).

7   Ibid.

8   Nosson Scherman, *Exodus 20, 8–11 Tanach, The Stone Edition, ArtScroll Series* (New York: Mesorah Publications Ltd., 1996).

9   Rabbi Chaim Miller, *Genesis 29:3, The Gutnick Edition* (New York: Kol Menachem, 2008).

10   Nosson Scherman, *Ezekiel 1, The Tanach, The Stone Edition, ArtScroll Series* (New York: Mesorah Publications Ltd., 1996).

11   Rabbi Yitzchak Ginsburgh, *The Hebrew Letters, Channels of Creative Consciousness* (Jerusalem: Gal Einai Publications, 1992).

12 Mesorah Publications, *Talmud Bavli, Schottenstein Edition* (New York: Mesorah Publications Ltd., 2000).

13 Rabbi Schneur Zalman, *Ethics of the Fathers, Siddur Tehillat Hashem, Annotated Edition,* trans. Nissan Mangel (Brooklyn: Merkos L'Inyonei Chinuch, Inc., 2002).

14 Shiva Rea, *Flow Yoga for Beginners,* directed by James Wvinner (Los Angeles: eOne Films, 2008), DVD.

15 Nissan Mindel, *Introduction, As for ME, My Prayer* (New York: Merkos L'Inyonei Chinuch, Inc., 1975).

16 Mesorah Publications, *Talmud Bavli, Schottenstein Edition* (New York: Mesorah Publications Ltd., 1995), Shabbat 31a.

17 Rabbi Menachem M. Schneerson, *Hayom Yom, "From Day to Day"* (New York: Otzar Hachassidim Lubavitch, 1988).

18 Rabbi Schneur Zalman, *Ethics of the Fathers, Siddur Tehillat Hashem, Annotated Edition,* trans. Nissan Mangel (New York: Merkos L'Inyonei Chinuch, Inc., 2002), chapter 2, section 4.

19 Rabbi Chaim Miller, *Genesis, 1:1, The Gutnick Edition* (New York: Kol Menachem, 2008).

20 Midrash Rabbah, *Genesis,* Vols. 1–2, trans H. Freedman and Maurice Simon (London: Soncino Press, 1983).

21 Mesorah Publications, *Talmud Bavli, Schottenstein Edition* (New York: Mesorah Publications Ltd., 1995).

22 Rabbi Chaim Miller, *Exodus 34, The Gutnick Edition* (New York: Kol Menachem, 2008).

23 Schneur Zalman of Liadi [the Alter Rebbe], *Tanya* (New York: Kehot Publication Society, 1984).

24 Rabbi Chaim Miller, *Genesis, 1:1, The Gutnick Edition* (New York: Kol Menachem, 2002), Genesis 2:21–22.

25 Mesorah Publications, *Talmud Bavli, Schottenstein Edition* (New York: Mesorah Publications Ltd., 1995).

26 Midrash Rabbah, *Genesis,* Vols. 1–2, trans. H. Freedman and Maurice Simon (London: Soncino Press, 1983), 18:2.

27 Rabbi Eliezer, *Midrash Pirkei d'Rabbi Eliezer*, trans. Gerald Friedlander (Skokie, IL: Varda Books, 2004), 8:2.

28 Midrash Rabbah, *Genesis*, Vols. 1–2, trans. H. Freedman and Maurice Simon (London: Soncino Press, 1983).

29 Rabbi Moshe Weissman, *Midrash Agada* (New York: Benei Yakov Publications, 1980).

Hebrew Letters Transliterated Chart

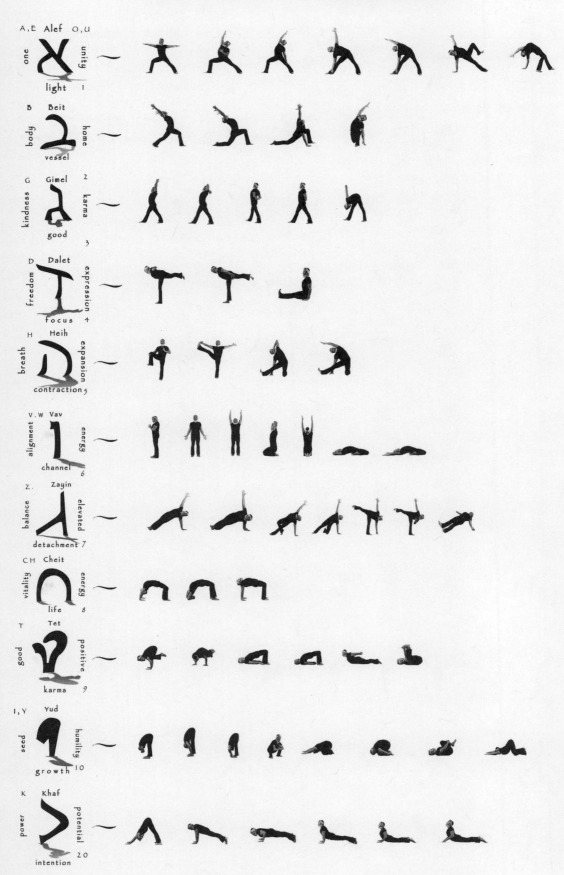

Hebrew Letters Transliterated Chart

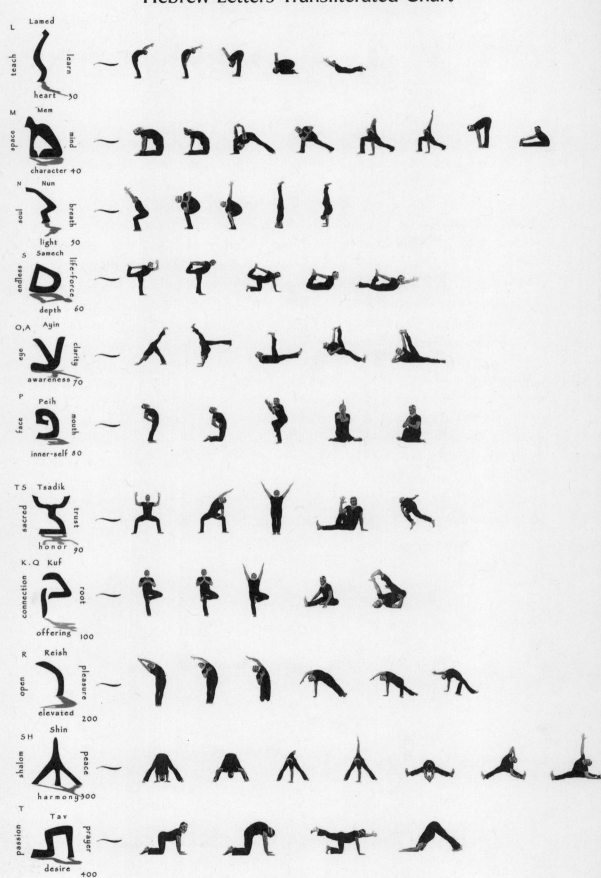

Yoga instructor, artist, spiritual teacher, author, attorney, and television host **Audi Gozlan, RYT,** has been a student of Kabalah for most of his life. At ten years old, he met his root spiritual teacher, the revered Lubavitcher Rebbe, and began to study in schools that taught mysticism in Canada and in the United States. Meditation came soon after, and he started incorporating the teachings of Kabalah into the practice of breathing. Audi then embraced yoga flow which led to the founding of Kabalah Yoga, a system of *hatha* flow yoga that fuses the ancient wisdom of Kabalah with the practice of yoga flow. Gozlan has been practicing yoga for more than seventeen years, and is a Prana Vinyasa teacher, as well as an assistant to Shiva Rea. He is producer of three Kabalah Yoga DVDs, and host of two popular television series in Canada, including the *Kabalah Yoga Show.*

Movement is life for foreword writer **Shiva Rea, MA,** a Prana Vinyasa teacher, activist, and innovator in the evolution of vinyasa yoga around the world. She is known for offering the synthesis form of vinyasa flow, bringing the roots of yoga alive for modern practitioners in creative, dynamic, and life-transforming ways for more than twenty-five years. She is a pioneer in reviving the art of *namaskar* through diverse *namaskars* or salutations; developing wave-sequencing, three-part vinyasa for energetic alignment; integrating the creative, spontaneous movement known as "sahaja" in postmodern yoga; and much more.

MORE BOOKS for the SPIRITUAL SEEKER

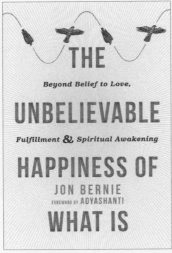

ISBN: 978-1626258716 | US $16.95

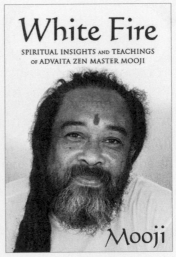

ISBN: 978-1684030583 | US $23.95

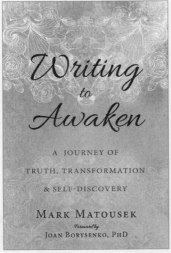

ISBN: 978-1626258686 | US $16.95

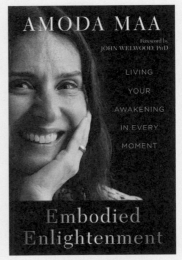

ISBN: 978-1626258396 | US $17.95

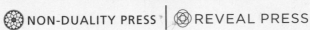